INTERNATIONAL REVIEWS ON NONYE TOCHI AGHANYA AND HER WORKS

Nonye Tochi Aghanya' s Think, Communicate, Heal: Discover the Healing Power of Clear Communication is a book which is a must read in the complex and involuted world order that we live in. Human life is complex. The technological boom has only helped in deepening the complex. In an age of auto correct and google search we have forgotten the art of thinking. In the milieu of instant messages and digital relationships we have forgotten the art of communication.

Nonye formulates a clear path on how to think and communicate better. The only difference that remains between technology and us is our ability to think and communicate. We can't lose these gifts. We need to learn the art of straight thinking and clear communication. This would make the world a better and much happier place.

Nonye transports us through myriad imageries and story lines to the power of effective thinking and communication which ultimately leads to healing hearts, building bridges and contented people all around.

Sarita Sharma PhD
Academician Author Poet Translator Keynote Speaker
Editor in Chief TAFFD's Magazine of the Future.

Browsing through Communication for health care as a practicing nurse on the internet, I came across the name "Nonye Tochi Aghanya." Realising she has written much on the subject with her deep knowledge, I got interested. Her most recent book Think, Communicate, heal: Discover the Healing Power of Clear Communication is what you don't get to see people talk about.

Here is the deal; the book focuses mainly on communication in the health care environment, says thinking and communicating make health care delivery better.

As a clinician (practicing registered nurse), I can't entirely agree less with Nonye's position because communication creates a wide range to help all health care workers to do their work effectively. Where there is a lack of communication, there is a breach in caregiving.

It is a truism that you can't just walk up to a patient and start administering medication without informed consent. It might lead to complexities as some patients may refuse anything you are to help on them.

For instance, I work in a hospital where if you don't communicate, you don't touch. First, you need to think, as the author posited here, you look at patient facial expressions to know how to communicate with this patient. Your thought process gives you an idea of how to go about it. Remember, not all patients like play.
As a nurse, I'm the active type, so I often have to think and observe the temperament or psychology of my patient before communicating.

Now we come down to communication. The ability to call patients by their names opens a room for that effective communication. It gives them a sense of belonging. When the patient replies/reacts/ as a healthcare provider, you have created a point of departure for a good communication process.
But where this is not established, it might be difficult for care and healing to be achieved.

The relationship between thinking, communication, and healing, keeps both the health facilities, healthcare workers, and the patients or clients in a healthy system of both body, mind, and spirit.

Conclusively, this book will help us solve a significant gap in our health care system, which is poor communication and thinking.

This book is a must-read for all health care providers/clinicians, and patients.

I am rating this book with a five star ✫

Uchendu Anastasia Chinenye
(A Registered Nurse in Nigeria)
I am currently working at Santa Antonio Medical Center, Agbara Ogun State, Nigeria.

I am a physician who has been in practice for over 20 years and I still found this book to be chock full of clinical pearls that I will definitely incorporate into my interations with patients. Ms Aghanya's insights about personality types and her witty and compassionate style made this book a pleasure to read. This book is a must read for anyone entering the healthcare profesiession as well as for seasoned clincians. Even lay people will find this book useful in understanding how clinicians tend to catagorize patients. In this age of limited time and resources, the proper clinician-patient relationship can make a world of difference. It's a fun read with lots of amusing cartoons, and you will definitely want to hold on to it as a reference.
Bill Song
The United States

After meeting Ms. Aghanya myself as a patient, I knew that she had a special gift for communicating with her patients. As she explains in her book, she not only has years of first-hand experience as a practitioner but learned as a patient as well, just how important proper communication and relationship building can be.
As I read her book, I learned a great deal about how I can better my relationship with my providers, as well as how I, as a hospital chaplain, can better interact with the patients who look to me as one of the members of their team of care providers. I strongly urge all healthcare providers as well as those who have found it difficult to develop trusting relationships with their providers to read this book.

James M Dakis
The United States

As a 30+ year nursing clinician, Nonye has written a wonderfully humorous, serious, and expertly crafted handbook for those who work in settings where communication is critical to good health/medical outcomes. I read this book in an hour or so. I enjoyed the story of her dad's non-compliance and how Nonye had to learn new ways to get 'on board' with him and his inner life, so he could get 'on board' with critical safety and health issues in his aging process.

I kept thinking the skills that Nonye passes on to the reader (e.g., nurses, doctors, etc.) really is a larger message about how to meet people 'where they are at'--to really listen deeply, and yet be authoritative when needed as well. I practiced many of these skills she lays out when I was a teacher and therapist, and now they are still important skills when being a father or husband or partner in a business. This is the bonus worth of her book--it is really for nearly everyone. She has concrete examples, with simple Do's and Don'ts. She knows what works in clinical settings with patients. I have no doubt about that.

At times I found myself wanting more detailed information about anxiety and fear, more in depth, more theory because these threads of emotional experience in the clinical setting she makes No. 1-- when it comes to being aware of what is going on as we encounter people who feel vulnerable (like a patient meeting a doctor for a consultation). Her idea of working in communication, as an authority figure, to attend and try to avoid "telling" people (clients, patients, partners) what to do, rather working on learning more about them and their situation before prescriptive discourses are used--is most critical, in my own experience as well. I think she is right to say most clinicians unrecognize their potential of creating fear/anxiety in people and that they unrecognize how that actually impacts cooperation with their patient (which, Nonye believes ought to be seen as a learning partnership). That's difficult advice to follow. Nonye, unfortunately with her pages of Do's and Don'ts and use of the words "should" and "must" --are to me quite unnecessary and reproduce the problem she is pointing out in good communications--that is, to avoid "telling" people what to do. This language in the book, I mentioned, is overly "telling" people what to do. So, even the best of us teaching about communication proficiency still have a lot to learn and we ought to pick our words carefully in what messages they convey about the nature of relationships. I think we can be more creative, and as Nonye says, number one value of a good practitioner in communications is to know yourself, listen to constructive feedback about how you communicate, and "Never stop learning" (as she says a few times in the book). I highly recommend this guidebook.

R. Michael Fisher
Founder and Lead Facilitator
The Fearology Institute, Canada

Here is an exciting book for all healthcare givers and a handbook for enhancing healthy living with evident instincts on the relationship between thinking and communication to heal.

I am most impressed on how the author systematically explained thoughts are produced, thinking and mindset, communication, and expression of ideas process, healing a manifestation of a communicated thought process.

It will interest me if the author would, in his subsequent publication, look at this work in the opposite direction " Think, communicate, hurt."

Having gone through the lines of this work, I am convinced that healthy living results from balanced thinking and communication. This book is a must-read for all healthcare givers, of which everyone is involved.

Rev. Sr. Maryann Chioma Okpala,
Nigeria

VIBRANT SHADES OF COMMUNICATION:

THINK, COMMUNICATE, HEAL: DISCOVER THE HEALING POWER OF CLEAR COMMUNICATION

Why talk about communication now, when we seem to communicate more than ever, across all social media platforms and devices? Everyone seems to be broadcasting, one way or another, for better or for worse. Pandemic has only emphasized our interdependence and dependence on communication, connection. But are we really conversing, connecting, are we really getting to know ourselves better, exchanging personal trust, thoughts and feelings, or are we simply enjoying the same memes, YouTubers, links, pics, filters, and whatever fits within an allowed number of characters? Or something in between?

The extent to which our life depends on meaningful, effective communication is most clearly, undeniably revealed in the medical setting. This is where Nonya Tochi Aghanya's takes us with her book *Think, Communicate, Heal: Discover the Healing Power of Clear Communication*

Communication starts even before leaving home, or we set foot in the doctor's office.

How do we decide which physician we can trust with our life? Do you find yourself listening to word of mouth and Google regarding doctor's clinical capabilities, checking their images, taking their gender, age, race, appearance into account? Once you do find a physician and surmount the challenge of scheduling an appointment any time soon in this post-pandemic world, once you actually do see the doctor, we'll often hear:

"Finally saw my doctor, and he gave me anti-depressants because I broke down crying while talking with him. He thought it was "just a menopause". Went to another doctor and got my blood work done. Turns out it was hyperthyroidism, and I also have some cervical issues".

"Finally saw my doctor, waited 52 minutes in the waiting room, and I swear he didn't spend more than 7 minutes with me! I looked at his notes in my chart: three sentences, three! I need to find me a new doctor!"

"Finally got my dog in to see the vet. There were so many dogs in the waiting room, so wild, by the time I got in to see the vet, I forgot what I was going to ask!"

Whatever the circumstances, clear thinking, good communication remains the key to greater health improvement.

Nonye Tochi Aghanya, MSc, RN, FNP-C, is uniquely qualified to guide us to the improvement of our meaningful, effective, compassionate communication skills. Her experiences as a Nigerian immigrant to the US, medical professional as well as patient, a wife, and mother of four daughters, an author, and keynote speaker have all contributed to the depth, proportions, and clarity of the mirror she holds up for us to observe and improve our current communication while at the same time weeding out our personal cognitive biases

"There are no defined rules for communicating effectively, but there are ways we can change lives and encourage growth by the things we say." ~ states Nonye Tochi Aghanya.

Nonya's new book "Think, Communicate, Heal: Discover the Healing Power of Clear Communication" is a natural progression of the previous four: Tips for Effective Communication; Principles for Improving Communication Anxiety and Improving Trust; Effective Communication: A Guidebook for Clinicians; Effective Communication: A Guidebook for Patients. Nonya starts by defining our body as a complex system of hosts in constant communication with each other, and ourselves.

Health is the system in a continuum, while the process of maintaining the balance within this continuum is where healthcare providers come in. Between the mental and physical aspects of our life, there is an essential process maintaining the integrity within the system: communication.

Nonye's book uses a transdisciplinary approach and storytelling to guide us on an educational walking tour of the relationship between thinking, communication, and healing. First, we visit Thinking and Mindset, where the relationship between thought, mindset, and communication is explored.

From there, we progress to Communication, where we explore the relationship between the thought process and verbal, as well as non-verbal expression. Lastly, we reach our destination: Healing - a manifestation of a communicated thought process.

The book argues that healing occurs in the balance between thinking and communication. It is intended to help everyone, in any setting, to understand the relationship between clear thinking, clear communication, and integral healing. Once we think and feel more clearly, we'll communicate more compassionately and effectively, starting with that little voice inside our heart and mind, and then with all around us ~ what a wonderful world it will be, healing all that ails and divides us!

Profound thanks to Nonya Tochi Aghanya for devoting herself to revealing to us the importance of the art of true communication.

Aidá Cemalovic

USA

ABOUT THE AUTHOR

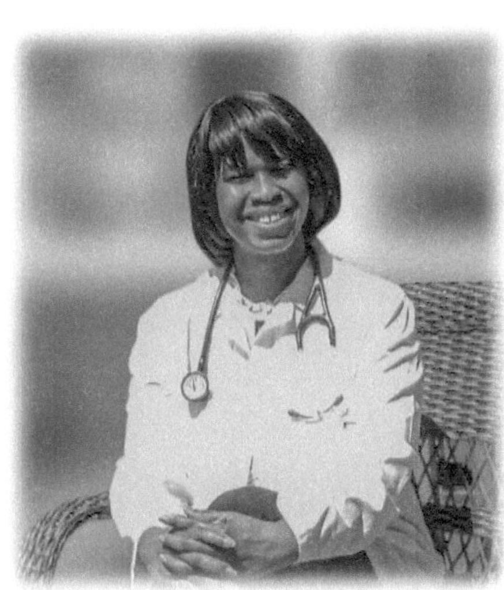

Nonye Tochi Aghanya MSc, RN, FNP-C obtained a Master of Science degree as a family nurse practitioner from Pace University, New York, and has worked in various outpatients/inpatient/homecare health settings. A registered nurse for 10 years, she later became a family nurse practitioner, a position she has held for many years.

For seven years she co-owned a private medical clinic and currently works in retail clinic for over thirteen years. A fellow of the American College of Healthcare Trustees, she is married, has four daughters, and resides with her family in Virginia.

THINK

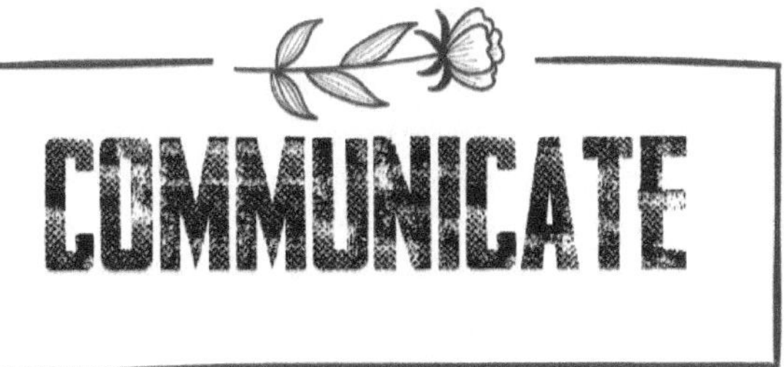

COMMUNICATE

HEAL

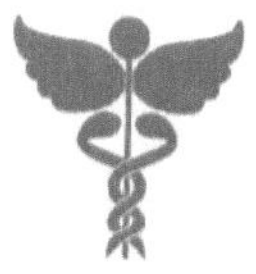

NONYE TOCHI AGHANYA

MSC, RN, FNP-C

EDITED BY UGO CHUKWU

THINK, COMMUNICATE, HEAL: DISCOVER THE DEALING POWER OF COMMUNICATION

ISBN: 9798535925936

Imprint: Published by TAFFD's Publishers.

TAFFD's Publishers titles may be purchased in bulk for educational, business, fund-raising, or sales promotional use. For information please email info@taffdspublisher.com

TO MY PARENTS: LATE ENGR. E. O.
AGHANYA AND MRS. C. AGHANYA.

"CHUKWU GOZIE EZIGBO NNE NA NNA
OMA M" (GOD BLESS MY GOOD PARENTS)

FOREWORD

The healthcare system has over the years advanced in leaps and bounds in almost all aspects of patient care, apart from one area – communication. The story that changes history begins with one person and one day. For healthcare and communication, it began in 1992 when Nonye Tochi Aghanya stepped into Dewitt Nursing Home in Brooklyn New York, and began her practice as a healthcare provider. What thereafter is the result of what you're about to experience in this book. The evidence and show of 30-year mastery in the patient-clinician relationship via communication.

Having read so much and followed the works of Nonye as an independent researcher, and encountering her works on the

World Fearlessness Movement NING, I was pleased to be invited by her to write this foreword.

In recent times I have been working closely with the author in understanding the place of communication in the healthcare niche. These led me to touch base with her other interconnected books, *Effective Communication: A GuideBook for Patients* and *Effective Communication: A Guide Book for Clinicians*. These guide books are heavily influenced by her first book - *Tips for Effective Communication: A Vital Tool for Trust Development in Healthcare*, which helps in making sense of this book THINK, COMMUNICATE, HEAL: Discover the Power of Clear Communication.

This three-part book teaches healthcare providers how to make sense of communication to pursue effective and efficient healing.

The author puts it this way; "our body is a complex system of multi-varied hosts in constant communication with each other. Maintaining a balanced and healthy life requires a lot of

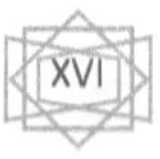

factors to be brought together. Health is a system in a continuum."

The essence of life is growth within this continuum. The task of every viable system is to maintain equilibrium within the vortex of this continuum. The process of maintaining balance within this continuum is the function of any healthcare provider. Balance within any healthy system begins from the mind down to the body. Between the mental and the physical, there is an essential process that maintains integrity within the system - this is communication.

This book is a must-have for all healthcare practitioners/providers, schools, and colleges of medical practices and should be kept in all clinics. Happy reading!

OSINAKACHI AKUMA KALU

Fearism Award-Winning Author & Speaker| Founder TAFFD's| Singularitarian|Futurist.

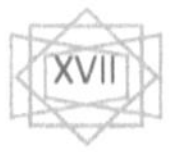

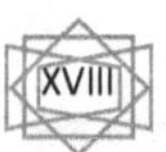

ACKNOWLEDGMENT

Understanding a particular reality doesn't happen in a vacuum but is seen through existential manifestation.

I want to thank all the patients I've encountered in the past thirty years for their diverse presentations that birth the various life-saving teaching styles of clinical practices.

A special thank you to Osinakachi Akuma Kalu, Desh Subba, and Michael Fisher for their supportive and excellent work in Fearism Studies. I am grateful to my friends on LinkedIn for their sincere engagements, constant encouragement, and well wishes.

Eunice Ifeanyichukwu

Evans Onyido

Jerin Hossain

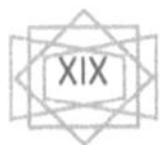

Jose Vasconcelos

Anne Levey

Ruth Amos

Zahmoul El Mays

Nesli N. Girgin

Antonio R. Freitas

Raj Raj

Pamela Leyvar

Frank N. Olson

And so many more friends, too numerous to mention.

To my siblings, you rock. Thank you for your patience and undying love.

I can't forget my readership and audience who constantly review, comment and critique my works; I say thank you for contributing to shaping my ideas. To all those whose works played vital roles as research materials, I say thank you.

Grateful Heart.

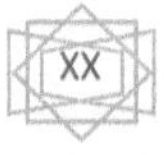

CONTENTS

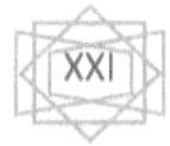

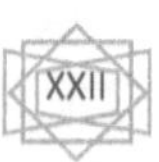

XXII

NOTE TO THE READER

Let me begin by thanking you for picking up this book to read. Change begins with one person and transformation happens one mind at a time. By reading this book you have made yourself a messenger of positive change and an active force for good in the world. I have written this book because I believe in the positive change educating minds like yours can bring to the world. My career and life have been in small healthcare spaces and within the 30 years it has spanned I have had the opportunity to help a few persons I have met as a healthcare provider. But I believe that by speaking to many people through this book I can impact a lot more lives. And so even though I might not have met you before, I pray our meeting will bear a fruit that would bring health, fulfillment, and peace in not just your life but those around you. I believe this book will impact you in great ways.

I would like to hear from you after you have read this book. You can write me at info@nonyetochi.com Feel free to share your testimonies of how this book has impacted your life and those around you. I encourage you also to gift a copy of this book to the people you care most about. Together we can create a healthy culture built on love, understanding, and effective communication. Life begins with communication and ends in its absence, burn the candle of life in your family, community, and workplace by keeping the knowledge and freedom that comes with effective communication. Leave a legacy by thinking clearly, communicating effectively, and healing holistically.

You can visit my website at www.nonyetochi.com to learn about my 30-year journey to effective communication. There you'll also find my other books, guidebooks, and courses where I share tips for effective communication.

I have an upcoming program called self-authoring suite for effective communication, this year 2021. This program offers you a chance to practice all the principles I have laid out in this book. You have the opportunity to take a journey like me, go within yourself, rediscover your power of communication and take charge of your internal monologue. By doing this you learn to express your thoughts more effectively so that your thoughts, words, and actions can be powerful enough to create results in the world. Effective communication is beyond learning how to talk. It's about commanding the forces within you and others to create a favorable outcome. Healing begins in the mind, as you learn in this book. The program will show you how to manifest it.

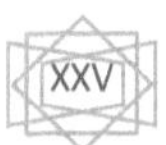

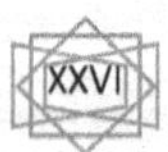

Introduction

Our body is a complex system of multi-varied hosts in constant communication with each other. Maintaining a balanced and healthy life requires a lot of factors to be brought together. Health is a system in a continuum. The essence of life is growth within this continuum. The task of every viable system is to maintain equilibrium within the vortex of this continuum. The process of maintaining balance within this continuum is the function of any healthcare provider. Balance within any healthy system begins from the mind down to the body. Between the mental and the physical, there is an essential process that maintains integrity within the system - this is communication.

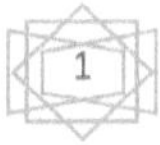

This book analyzes the relationship between thinking, communication, and healing - as the 3-part process that brings about a healthy system in any person. Using a transdisciplinary approach, it explores the disciplines of psychology, neuroscience, neuro-linguistic programming (NLP) philosophy of language, linguistics, biology, and health science.

The main thesis is thus:

- Thought produces thinking and mindset

- Communication is an expression of thought process

- Healing is a manifestation of a communicated thought process.

The book using the narrative tool of storytelling takes the reader on an educational and revelatory journey to see the relationship between thinking, communication, and healing. It introduces the concept of the *healthcare giver* as the responsibility of the healthcare provider. It helps the patient to see the relationship between her thinking and her communication to help her understand that healing is the consequence of these two

This book is intended to help people within and outside the healthcare environment to understand the relationship between clear thinking, clear communication, and integral healing of a person.

Communication is life, thinking is the progenesis, healthcare is where it begins.

The book is divided into three parts

1. **Thinking and Mindset** - where I explore the relationship between thought, mindset, and communication. It offers principles, strategies, and approaches for maintaining a healthy mindset that is essential to good health.

2. **Communication** - where I explore the relationship between thought process and expression (verbal and

non-verbal) offering strategies and principles for effective communication.

3. **Healing** - where I explore how the relationship between thought and mindset, generates healing as the final part of restoration. Here the book argues that without balance between thinking and communication healing that results in healthcare cannot occur.

As you read through these pages, may you be inspired by truth and healed by the changing of your mind.

PART ONE

THINK

Communication begins in the mind. It begins with the energy of a single spark of thought. This understanding is at the heart of every great feat that has been achieved in the world. From the creation of ampicillin to the setting of the first man on the moon. Thought can bear positive energy or negative energy, depending on the source and nature of its organization. Health is a communicated thought process. Every thought creates the signature tone that the cells in the body adopt as instructions for ordering our tissues and organs. To take charge of your health you must learn to take charge of your thoughts. This is an art to be learned, it is not given naturally. Taking charge of your thoughts begins with understanding how your mind works. Nature has given you some mental latitude to control what happens in your mind through your internal monologue. If you must take charge of your thoughts, you must learn how to manage and utilize your internal monologue.

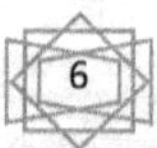

CHAPTER ONE

TRAPPED IN HIS BODY

What would you do if you were locked in your body, your brain intact but with no way to communicate? How do you survive emotionally when you are invisible to everyone you know and love?

It was in the late '80s, and young Martin Pistorius, growing up in South Africa, was mostly thinking about electronics, resistors, and transistors and you name it.

But at age 12, his life took an unexpected turn. He came down with a strange illness. The doctors weren't sure what it was, but their best guess was cryptococcal meningitis. He got

progressively worse. Eventually, he lost his ability to move by himself, his ability to make eye contact, and finally, his ability to speak. His parents, Rodney and Joan Pistorius were told that he was as good as not there, a vegetable. The hospital told them to take him home and keep him comfortable until he died.

But after one month he didn't die, then one month turned to one year, and then two, three, four. "Martin just kept going, just kept going," his mother says. His father would get up at 5 o'clock in the morning, get him dressed, load him in the car, take him to the special care center where he'd leave him. "Eight hours later, I'd pick him up, bathe him, feed him, put him in bed, set my alarm for two hours so that I'd wake up to turn him so that he didn't get bedsores," Rodney, his father recalls.

That was their life, for 12 years. Joan vividly remembers looking at Martin one day and saying: " 'I hope you die.' I know that's a horrible thing to say, I just wanted some sort of relief.

"And she didn't think her son was there to hear it. But he was.

"Yes, I was there, not from the very beginning, but about two years into my vegetative state, I began to wake up," says Martin, now age 39 and living in Harlow, England. He thinks he began to wake up when he was 14 or 15 years old. "I was aware of everything, just like any normal person," Martin says.

But although he could see and understand everything, he couldn't move his body. "Everyone was so used to me not being there that they didn't notice when I began to be present again," he says. "The stark reality hit me that I was going to spend the rest of my life like that — totally alone."

He was trapped, with only his thoughts for company. And they weren't particularly nice thoughts. "No one will ever show me tenderness. No one will ever love me. And of course there was no way to escape," he thought, "You are doomed."

So he figured his only option was to leave his thoughts behind. That was his first strategy — disengaging his thoughts — and he says he got really good at it. "You don't really think about anything," Martin says. "You simply exist. It's a very dark place to find yourself because, in a sense, you are allowing yourself to vanish."

But occasionally there were things that elicited thoughts he could not ignore. Like Barney. "I cannot even express to you how much I hated Barney," Martin says. "I often spent my days positioned in front of the TV watching Barney reruns. I think because Barney is so happy and jolly, and I absolutely wasn't"

Then one day, he decided he'd had enough. He wanted to gain some small measure of control over his day. So he figured out how to tell time by how the sun moved across a room. That was the start. And to do this, he needed to know what time it was because if he could know what time it was, he could know when it would end and, specifically, how much closer he was to his favorite moment in the day.

Now, the problem was that Martin was rarely seated near a clock. So he calls upon these old allies - these thoughts - to help him carefully study the lengths of the shadows. "I would watch how the sun moved across the room or how a shadow moved throughout the day." Martin explains. And he begins to match what he sees with little bits of information he's able to collect - what he hears on the television, a radio report, a nurse mentioning the time. It was a puzzle to solve, and he did it. Within a few months, he could read the shadows like a clock.

He could tell the time of day by the shadows. It was his first semblance of control. Simply knowing where he was in the day gave him the sense of being able to climb through it. And this experience ultimately led him to start thinking about his thoughts differently. As Martin puts it "I think your thoughts are integrated - connected and part of you." He realized that they could help him, and so he started listening to them again.

"I'd have conversations with myself and other people in my head." And if a particularly dark thought came up...You are pathetic, powerless. He'd try to contend with it. Like one time, shortly after having the drool wiped from his chin by a nurse. He said to Martin, "You are pathetic."

He happened to notice a song playing on the radio. Whitney Houston was singing the "Greatest Love of All." In the song, she says, no matter what they take from me, they can't take away my dignity. "I sat there and thought, you want to bet?" He remembers.

The point is reengaging with his thoughts transformed his world. Life began to have purpose.

As Martin recounts. "I would literally live in my imagination, sometimes to such an extent that I became oblivious to my surroundings." Which you know could be rough.

Eventually, Martin found a way to reframe even the ugliest thoughts that haunted him. Like when his mother said, "I hope you die." "The rest of the world felt so far away when she said those words," Martin recalls.

But he began to wrestle with it. Why would a mother say that?

"As time passed, I gradually learned to understand my mother's desperation. Every time she looked at me, she could see only a cruel parody of the once-healthy child she had loved so much," which actually made him feel closer to her. And so onward he went, trying now to understand his dark thoughts instead of just ignoring them all, which brings us to the last act of his story - the way in which Martin is able to climb out.

And slowly, as his mind felt better, something else happened — his body began to get better, too. It involved inexplicable neurological developments and a painstaking battle to prove that he existed.

Martin slowly regained some control of his body. By the time he was in his mid-20s, he could squeeze your hand on occasion. And he was getting better and better at holding himself upright in his chair. Now, the doctors told his parents that he still had the intelligence level of a 3-month-old baby. But one nurse named Verna, an aromatherapist began coming to the care home about once a week. She was convinced that there was something there. And so she eventually convinced his parents to get Martin reassessed at another medical center. "She urged my parents to have me tested by experts in augmentative and alternative communication". There, he was given a test where he had to identify different objects by pointing at them with his eyes. And he passed, not with flying colors, but he passed. And within a year, he was beginning to use a computer program to communicate. Joan, who came home to care for Martin, help him with his physical therapy, and most importantly, purchase this kind of joystick for the computer. "A proximity switch, which is just something that you knocked," he explains.

And though it took him about a year to get the hang of it. Once he did, everything changed because suddenly he had a way to select the words he wanted to say. He could say "I am cold. I am hungry. I want toast." And as words came back, gradually, so did other things. He started moving his eyes and moving his head and almost nodding, asking for coffee by stirring his hands around and things like that.

Within two years of passing that assessment test, Martin gets a job filing papers at a local government office. As Martin explained, "I wanted to prove that I could do more than just speak words via a laptop."

Around this time, his nurse savior Verna mentioned she's having trouble with her computer. And Martin, who has not tinkered with electronics since he was 12 years old, fixes it.

After that, he scraps the government job and starts a web design company. He gets into college to study computer science. He writes a book. He learns how to drive. "Martin achieves everything he wants to do." His Mum says.

As his wife, Joanna explains, "When Martin talks about me or types about me, he always starts smiling". Joanna was a friend of Martin's sister. And the two of them first met over Skype.

"I was a manager for the social work team for a hospital social work team". Joanna said it was the honesty with which he expressed his thoughts that drew her to Martin. They got married in 2009. Martin was 33 years old.

Narrating his life experience, Martin explains on a TedX talk

> "Communication is what makes us human, enabling us to connect on the deepest level with those around us -- telling our own stories, expressing wants, needs, and desires, or hearing those of others by really listening. All this is how the world knows who we are. So who are we without it?... True communication increases understanding and creates a more caring and compassionate world. Once, I was perceived to be an inanimate object, a mindless phantom of a boy in a wheelchair. Today, I am so much more. A husband, a son, a friend, a brother, a business owner, a first-class honors graduate, a keen amateur photographer. It is my ability to communicate that has given me all this...Our words, however we communicate them, are just as powerful. Whether we speak the words with our own voices, type them with our eyes, or communicate them non-verbally to someone who speaks them for us, words are among our most powerful tools. I have come to you through a

terrible darkness, pulled from it by caring souls and by language itself. The act of you listening to me today brings me farther into the light. We are shining here together. If there is one most difficult obstacle to my way of communicating, it is that sometimes I want to shout and other times simply to whisper a word of love or gratitude. It all sounds the same.

I began to communicate more, I realized that it was in fact only just the beginning of creating a new voice for myself. I was thrust into a world I didn't quite know how to function in.... realized that some people would only listen to me if what I said was in line with what they expected. Otherwise, it was disregarded and they did what they felt was best. I discovered that true communication is about more than merely physically conveying a message. It is about getting the message heard and respected."

As NPR'S narrator of the story, Lulu Miller, puts it: "So how is it that Martin has been able to achieve all this? Now, I don't want to oversimplify it because it was many things - Martin's naturally strong will, flukes of electricity in the brain, a really dedicated family. But I do think that his decision to lean back into those thoughts way back when, instead of just spending his life detaching, in some way helped him, in part because it probably kept his mind occupied and allowed him to emerge this kind of well-oiled machine of mental ability, but also because I think his leaning into those dark thoughts in particular gave him a kind of self-understanding and humor about the human condition that allowed him to snag the very best thing in his life."[1]

Thought and Energy

This part of the book has been addressed to both healthcare providers and non-healthcare providers.

What is thought? What is its function in us?

All our actions begin in thought. Thought is the primary place where a lot of things that happen in our lives begin. The idea to create begins as a thought. The idea to marry a spouse,

---

[1] Story adapted in full from NPR's podcast program "Invisiblia"

to buy a house, to buy a car, to start a business, the idea to live healthily or unhealthily, the idea to get sick and to heal, the idea to practically begin anything we do begins as a thought. Now this includes the idea to do or not to do anything, it equally includes the idea to live in a particular state or not to.

You see, thoughts are things and they are not just contents of the mind that we are conscious of, they equally include the ones we are unconscious about. A thought is simply a form of energy that inhabits the mind from where larger forms of energy like ideas and emotions are generated.

The prevalent form of energy that saturates the mind is the one that conditions the dominating form of energy that you feel as emotions. Emotions are thought signatures. They tell us the quality of our dominating thoughts - conscious or unconscious.

Health is the expression of the prevalent energy as a state of being - influenced by both internal and external stimuli. To a large extent our health is dependent to a large degree on the quality of energy you have in your body. Positive energy is a balancing of all the systems that make up your biology. Your cells and the immune system have been charged with this common task of maintaining balance within your body.

The task of maintaining an energy level that will create health begins in the thought. All energy generation begins first in the thought of your mind. Then it sets the tune for the cells of your body to create the tissues and organs in the body.

But what is the source of thoughts? According to Broadcast Engineer, Tamara Ivy Iverson, "At present, there is no known way to measure the energy of thought other than by measuring the brain with an electroencephalogram, (EEG), or a scan which shows where the brain is active under certain conditions...Since slight electrical currents are flowing, (picked up by the EEG), it might be possible to detect slight magnetic fields generated by thought with very sensitive equipment.

There are demonstrable effects on plants and even animals by "projecting" thoughts to them. For example, thinking "love" to one plant will cause it to grow faster while projecting "hate" towards another plant can cause it to stunt or even wither and die. This works over long distances, (more than a few yards), but the medium of transference is unknown.

Whilst this might not give us an exhaustive answer to the question we posed, it leaves us with a clue of where to find our answer - energy.

According to the learning coach Ugo Chukwu, our minds have a structure that is built based on ancestral memory. This is memory encoded into our DNA that conditions the disposition of our biology and psychology. The structure of the mind creates a mental framework that determines how you receive and process information. How do you determine what kinds of thoughts and ideas that pop into your mind? Well, the answer is that you don't, you can't because it's not your conscious mind that does that, it is the structure of your mind that does that. This is why two people will receive the same information but have different ideas of information. If the type of idea to be generated was dependent solely on the type of information they both received, then they would both come up with the same idea, but the difference shows that there's something else at stake that is beyond the information received. And that is the structure of their mind which determines the way the information is processed. Ugo Chukwu calls this intelligence. It is the level and nature of one's intelligence that determines how information is processed by the mind. This is perhaps how thought is generated. Ancestral memories encoded in your DNA (in the form of genetic information) sets the tone for the formation of both your biology and psychology. With the interaction of the environment, a mental framework is created. This determines the level and nature of your intelligence. This way your intelligence is created. Your mind will generate thought on its own and whenever it encounters information based on your intelligence or mental blueprint, and this will set the tone for the kind of energy that would be generated within your body. Energy is the blueprint of health in the body.

By thought, you can think yourself sick. You can equally think of yourself healthy. It all depends on which route you decide to take; it all depends on the consistent thought narrative that runs through your mind.

CHAPTER TWO –

INTERNAL MONOLOGUE AND PROCESSES

Thoughts exist on two levels - subconscious and conscious thoughts. Subconscious thoughts operate deep within the mind where you cannot control. It runs 95% of our daily activities. It is like the giant operating system within us. With vast memory storage and very huge processing power. The body delivers about 11 million bits of data for the brain to process. Of that total amount researchers have found that the conscious mind processes only about 40 to 50 bits of data per second based on variant available data. The subconscious mind can process 20 000 000 bits of info per second. So the subconscious mind can process 500,000 times more than the conscious mind is able to.

This according to Dr. Bruce Lipton, in his book "The Biology of Belief". There is no formal agreement on how fast the subconscious mind works. Researchers at the University of Pennsylvania School of Medicine estimate the human retina can transmit visual input at a rate of approximately 10 million bits per second. Consciousness is often assumed to be the dominant feature of the brain. According to data from emerging studies, it is now clear to us that most brain functions happen without our awareness and most bodily activities occur without conscious awareness.

Another study indicates that the subconscious mind processes 400 billion bits of information per second, and the impulses travel at a speed of 100,000 mph! This is in stark contrast to your conscious mind, which processes only about 2,000 bits of information per second and transmits impulses at only 100-150 mph. There are 50 trillion cells in our body performing trillions of processes, requiring a great deal of processing power. It is estimated that only about 0.01% of all brain activity is conscious. It is as if roughly 10'000 cinema films are playing simultaneously in the brain, but we are consciously aware of only one.

In total, the brain processes 320 Gb/s of data! With such a large amount of processing power, it can control a lot of your life.

Thoughts can exist both in the conscious and subconscious parts of your mind. When they exist in the conscious mind, you are aware of it, but you're often not aware of it when they exist in the subconscious. But this doesn't mean that it does not affect your life, it does. The only thing is that the effects happen on a subliminal level. Insignificant enough for you to understand how they control your life.

The mechanism of your subconscious mind is very useful in helping you function effectively as a human being even when it comes to your communication. The only problem is that we are oftentimes unaware of how it does it. Because of this, we are often at the mercy of its internal processes and communication even when they are designed against our wellbeing. We are born into an environment that we did not wish for. And as such, we pick cues from it that form our subconscious programming without the choice to do any of these.

Communication is a delicate art that begins first in the internal processes of the mind. Our verbal expressions are simply communicated thoughts that have been magnified. But more than anything else your internal energy system determines the state of your health and wellbeing. Thoughts as the contents of our minds control our internal energy system and therefore, our health to a large extent. Within the deep recesses of your mind is an internal communication system that begins with thoughts and multiplies into other things like ideas and mindset that determines what happens in your life.

According to psychologists, the subconscious mind becomes shaped and hard-pressed after the age of seven, some other estimates put it at thirteen.

But whatever be the case, neuroscience makes us understand that in processing information your whole brain is fully engaged. According to Robert M Sapolsky, a Neuroendocrinologist, Professor of Biology, and Neurology at Stanford University "The human brain isn't fully developed until 25 years of age. Everything's there except for the frontal cortex, which is the last thing to mature. An immature frontal cortex explains the spectrum of teenage behaviors: it's what makes adolescents adolescent. Meaning that at a very young age your subconscious mind, the area that controls 95% of your internal communication system is formed. It means you don't have much control over what kind of information structures your mind and shapes your personality, including your communicative abilities. Starting from your thought processes to your speech mannerism. If this internal communication system is not set with your consent, it, therefore, means that it may contain most things that might not be serving your interest. Things such as your lifestyle and wellbeing.

If you are going to take charge of your life, you have to exercise considerable control over your internal processes. This is where internal monologue comes in as a means of taking charge of your internal communication process.

Internal monologue is the internal communicative processing system where subconscious thoughts come into the rearview so that you can access and analyze them. It comes in the form of that little voice in your head that talks all the time nonstop. The one you use to analyze, dissect and synthesize your thoughts and ideas before you verbalize or act on them.

This inner monologue is a very useful system in regulating the nature and quality of thought that pop up now and again in your mind. Nature has designed it in such a way that since you don't have direct access to your subconscious mind which has structured your mind, determining what kind of thoughts to pop up, you can access these thoughts and change them before they have the opportunity to get out in any form of expression. This is where your conscious mind kicks in with its processing capability. The conscious mind uses internal monologue as an internal regulating system that checks and balances thoughts and feelings. It analyzes its usefulness to you and judges the best action to take based on your needs and goals. It equally allows you to run mental simulations with which you can use to process actions before you engage in them.

The interesting thing about your internal monologue is that it gives you the ability to restructure your subconscious mind after the needed effort and work.

Your mind can access the nature and quality of thoughts that predominate your internal thought communication, based on your constant emotions. Emotions are the language of the subconscious mind. Once you can feel it, the thought exists in your mind. It's only waiting for maturation. However, your system is set in such a way that when that feeling kicks in, your conscious processing systems turn on your internal monologue system to allow you to use language to process the information contained in the emotions that are being generated. This is where you have the chance to change things and create a new thought and mindset that will set the tone for your communications and health.

When you have that feeling and that voice comes up in your head, what you say in those moments determines it all. As you communicate with yourself, you begin to shape your internal communication system. The words you use and what those words mean for you in these moments matter a lot. This is because at best, words are the signature tones in which feelings and emotions are translated. When you feel those emotions and you translate them into words you create an internal language for yourself. Your internal language acts as feedback to your subconscious mind. It sends back a command response asking it to change program settings that are not in alignment. If the thoughts in the subconscious mind are producing negative language and your internal monologue "rewords" your internal language system to be positive, over time it will send feedback to the subconscious mind to change the tone of its thoughts to positive.

It is during your internal monologue that your subconscious pattern becomes visible to assessment and readjustment. It's like you are being offered an opportunity to make some changes before the final settings go into action to set the tone for your health.

This is what Martin in our story applied as the first step of engaging his thoughts and conquering the negative thought patterns that hunted his mind. By using his internal monologue to access his thoughts, he began to take charge of his inner communication. This was the thing that set the stage for his healing process and transformation. By learning how to master his inner language through internal monologue, first, before speaking, he prepared himself to become an effective communicator. His wife confessed to the fact that the first time she discussed with him she immediately liked him because of how honest he was in the answers he gave her. But even more importantly, how well he had taken time to understand human nature. It, therefore, goes to say that the oldest advice in the book "Man know thyself" begins with mastering your internal monologue. For if you can control what happens inside, you have already mastered what's going to happen outside.

Educating the Language of Your Internal Monologue.

You have learned that your internal monologue offers you the chance to make changes in the nature and quality of thoughts your unknown mind (subconscious mind) produces. Now the more important question is, how do you do it?

The greatest power that we have been endowed with as a species, is the ability to learn, unlearn and relearn. This capacity offers you the ability to make changes to your ever-changing world.

Using your learning capability, you can educate your internal monologue. Just like you can set the language of your phone to a particular language. You can set your internal language to a particular emotional language that reflects the kind of life you want for yourself. The way you do this is by exercising control over these three things: Words, belief, and needs.

The Right Words: It is estimated that human beings first evolved language around 50,000–150,000 years ago, which is around the time when modern Homo sapiens evolved. Other researchers estimate that since our prefrontal cortex plays a pivotal role in our use of language it is most probable that we developed language at the same time that we developed this part of our brains that provides the executive functions of our brain. Following the evolution of the PFC, we invented language, and with it came free will - the ability to choose.

Words, though not perfect, are nonetheless powerful vehicles for communicating thoughts and emotions. When you understand the power of words and educate yourself in its usage you equip yourself with one of the most powerful tools of life. As the German philosopher Wittgenstein correctly says: "The limits of my language mean the limits of my world.", and in addition, I say both internal and external language. You first set your internal language before you express your external language. Your external language is an expression of your internal language.

If you understand this, then you understand how you can literally think yourself sick by merely repeating bad thoughts in your head. The quality of the words you use and the meaning of the words for you determines the feelings they will generate in you.

Educating your internal monologue begins with building the vocabulary and imbuing those words with the meanings that have useful significance for you. We live in a world and culture that most times use words without a deep understanding of their meaning. This comes at a great cost, for words misunderstood means principles misapplied. With a clear understanding of words comes a vivid interpretation of experiences. If you can properly interpret your experiences and store their memories in your mind with the proper words, then you can develop considerable control over your life.

For most people, their vocabulary is not built by them, but by their associations and society. We adopt the meaning of words based on their common usage in our specific culture. Though this might seem inevitable as we are born into a society and we learn our mother tongue as we observe our parents and other speakers, but we can still rewrite this through study, research and reflection. By doing this you build a repertoire of words and their meaning, which will help you begin to take charge of your internal monologue.

Secondly, you need to educate your internal monologue by determining what kind of words you use regularly on yourself.

These words are super important because as you use them more and more in your head, they begin to form the language of your verbal expressions. What you hear from people comes from the abundance of their hearts. By educating yourself through study, research, and reflection, the words you create from these experiences will begin to inebriate your heart and mind. Those words will affect your thinking now and always.

Believe the Words You Speak to Yourself. A belief is an idea one accepts as being true or real. Thoughts generate energy and organize themselves into an intelligent unit called ideas. When these ideas as contents of your mind begin to take root in your thinking, they hijack your cognitive structures and begin to produce feelings of certainty in you. A dopaminergic reaction motivates them to act based on the contents or knowledge that back your belief. What this means, therefore, is that belief is any cognitive content held as true. Ugo Chukwu defines it well when he summarized it as " a feeling of certainty that makes you accept something as true".

When you accept the words that you use in your internal monologue as true and it produces a feeling of certainty, then know at that point you have successfully rewired the language of your subconscious mind.

The real catch is that any message you repeat long enough in your internal monologue will lock itself as emotion and produce a sensation whenever you think about it or say the words. This is why you must ensure that you follow the next step.

Vigilance: This is a very important factor when it comes to setting your internal language. As Thomas Jefferson acknowledges: "The price of freedom is eternal vigilance." If you want to take charge of your internal monologue, then you must commit yourself to be an active watchdog over the kinds of thoughts that pop up in your mind always. Since you don't control how these thoughts pop up, you might as well control your thinking when they do.

Two key skills that will help you to do this are metacognition and meditation.

With meditation, you learn how to notice and monitor the contents of your mind by monitoring your thoughts and the feelings they produce. Research shows that mediation trains the areas of your brain that are tasked with controlling your emotions - the amygdala. Mental vigilance is a buildable muscle that you train with practice. As you practice every day, you develop the ability to become more conscious of your thoughts and emotions. This is a very powerful tool in helping prevent disease, inducing healing, and communicating effectively.

The second is the skill of metacognition. Which gives you the ability to think about your thinking. Metacognition is an awareness of one's thought processes and an understanding of the patterns behind them. The term comes from the root word "meta" which means beyond and or on top of - thinking. When you think about eating and you think about why you are thinking about eating, that is metacognition. This skill can be deployed in many ways to monitor your thought processes.

Vigilance is an important factor when it comes to taking charge of your internal language and setting the tone for internal monologue and health.

The Story of Mary

Mary, not her real name, is a young girl from Abia State. She comes from a devoted Catholic background that emphasizes the importance of chastity and the need for young girls to remain virgins until marriage. Her dad was very active in church services. He was a catechist in the church. Moreover, her mother served as the women's leader in her parish. The family had close relations with the priests. In church, the priests communicated to Mary and her parents the importance of adhering to the morals of the church. A life the family strived to live up to. The family had two daughters Caroline and Mary. Mary was the second.

Mary belonged to a pious group in the church called Mary League, a group that promoted the virtues ascribed to the biblical Christian Mary the mother of Jesus. The group prohibited young girls from wearing trousers, having boyfriends, or seeing any man before marriage. Mary equally sang in the choir which had an organized practice of shaming young girls who got pregnant out of wedlock. And so Mary's life was inspired by the moral rules of the church. Mary is Igbo and in her native culture sex was regarded as a shameful thing. In her village women were asked to cover their bodies so that men would not see their bodies. A woman that gets pregnant before marriage is shamed and her family fined for humiliating the kindred and community.

Soon Mary started witnessing puberty. At 14 she started noticing changes in her body and with that boys started coming closer. She liked how she felt when a boy touches her or when she sees a love scene in a movie, but just after feeling that way she immediately feels remorse and shame for how she felt.

At 16 Mary had a boyfriend. One evening she was chatting with the boy over the phone unknown to her that her mum was eavesdropping on her call. After the call, the mom called her in and sounded a stern warning to her: "If you ever get pregnant in this house you're on your own". Her words scared Mary. She was terrified at the thought of getting pregnant. So she vowed within herself never to fall into such a thing. According to Mary, she said these words in her head: "I will show mom that I will never get pregnant". Mary would remind herself of these words whenever any man approached her for a relationship. Or whenever the thoughts of sex pop up in her mind.

Eight years later, Mary was finally ready to be with a man and she got happily married to Phillip. Her husband, Philip, was so eager to be with Mary because she was a virgin. And based on their tradition marrying a virgin was a thing of honor to the man, and respect for the wife. Her family basked in the euphoria of the honor and respect Mary's marriage and her virginity had brought upon the family. Immediately, after their wedding, the couple went on a much-fantasized honeymoon in Calabar, where they planned to consummate their love. Mary was equally excited as her husband. They are both to have sex for the first time after so many years of chastity and abstinence.

But to the utter disappointment of the couple when they got in bed to consummate their love, they were unable to have sex. Mary was so terrified of the experience that she got out of bed crying. The husband consoled and assured her that she would get over it with time. They both thought it was a result of fear of the first experience. But their assumptions soon turned out to be wrong. They tried the next day and it failed, and the third day, and it went from a week to a month to a year. The husband was both surprised and frustrated. Mary was depressed and devastated. The marriage began to suffer the weight of the challenge.

The couple sought medical help at the hands of their private doctor who after examining Mary referred them to a gynecologist. When they met the gynecologist, she examined Mary and asked her a few questions. After which Mary was diagnosed with a medical condition known as vaginismus.

Vaginismus is a condition involving a muscle spasm in the pelvic floor muscles. It can make it painful, difficult, or impossible for a woman to have sexual intercourse, undergo a gynecological exam, and insert a tampon in the vagina. When she tries to insert an object such as a tampon, penis, or speculum into the vagina, it becomes tightened due to an involuntary contraction of the pelvic floor muscles. This leads to generalized muscle spasms, pain, and temporary cessation of breathing.

This condition can be caused by many issues that range from psychological to physical. Some women develop vaginismus after menopause. When estrogen levels drop, a lack of vaginal lubrication and elasticity makes intercourse painful, stressful, or impossible. Other times the leading causes could be psychological as in past sexual abuse or trauma, past painful intercourse, emotional factors, and trauma caused by past impressions about sex. In Mary's case, the latter was the case. Her internal monologue conditioned by culture and the opinions of others caused a psychological trauma that created her condition.

How we think and communicate within ourselves contributes a lot to our mental state which practically controls every other aspect of our lives. Using our internal monologue, we can take charge of our thought patterns and create the kind of reality we want for ourselves.

CHAPTER THREE –

MIND AND BODY

The mind is the seat of consciousness where thoughts begin, are organized and the energy frequency of these thoughts formulated and sent out. The power of the mind in formulating thoughts and controlling the body cannot be underestimated.

When you look at yourself in the mirror what do you see? You probably say I see myself, I see me. You think of yourself as a single entity with a single body. But that is wrong. On the contrary, when you look at the mirror you are not seeing an individual you. You are looking at trillions of entities swimming around and vibrating at a high speed to create structure, system, and organization that the senses can perceive as a body. These entities are cells and on their own they have intelligence. Cells exist in two forms: unicellular and multicellular. Unicellular cells like amoeba exist on their own as single intelligent life forms. It organizes itself and operates in the world. However, entities like this don't survive as easily and pass on their genes to the next generation as their counterparts - the multicellular life forms.

Multicellular entities are a group of cells that come together to co-exist. They submit their individual intelligence and then take on a central intelligence system that allows them to self-organize. This enables them to survive easily and pass on their genes to the next generation. Cells that come together to co-exist as one entity, share something important - their energy vibration is the same. And so they come together and based on their energy level that vibrates at the same frequency to create harmony. This is an essential element in any system - the establishment of equilibrium and order. When this exists there is health. In its absence, there's a lack of integrity and chaos that results in sickness.

Humans are complex organisms made up of trillions of cells, each with its own structure and function. Scientists have come a long way in estimating the number of cells in the average human body. Most recent estimates put the number of cells at around 30 trillion.

With over thirty trillion cells swirling around and going about their businesses, there's bound to be chaos and disharmony if not checked, because each cell is independently intelligent. How then do we get the level of order and effective cooperation we have between the cells in our bodies? That's because the cells have submitted their individual autonomy to a central authority in the body to manage all the processes in the system and respect any order that has been given by this central authority--the brain. The brain is the central processing unit in the human system. It is where information is processed and order sent out to different parts of the body.

The brain controls what you think and feel, how you learn and remember, and the way you move and talk. But it also controls things you're less aware of — like the beating of your heart and the digestion of your food. Think of the brain as a central computer that controls all the body's functions. Take for example the Medulla Oblongata.- the structure is caudal - it is part of the brain stem, between the pons and spinal cord. It is responsible for maintaining vital body functions, such as breathing, digestion, and heartbeat. And these functions are unconscious and involuntary. This means the brain is in charge of the functions that we are unaware of. It is indeed the central processing unit of the body. All the cells in other parts of the body take instructions from it. This is really interesting to think about. If the brain tells the cells in your body to produce hormones for digesting food, they do. If it tells them to produce hormones to manage pregnancy for women, it does. When you get injured, you feel the pain because your brain tells your body to send you signals of pain to the degree of the damage that has been done to your tissues, so that you cooperate with it in helping you heal. But this isn't where it ends. If the brain equally tells the cells in your body to die, they would also obey that instruction.

We know of apoptosis. The death of cells occurs as a normal and controlled part of an organism's growth or development. Also in the case of cancer what happens is an overgrowth of cells making them cancerous. And in the case of Hypoplasia, there's an undergrowth of cells causing incomplete development of a tissue or organ.

Clearly what this tells us is that our brains can communicate life or death to the cells in our brain.

But the brain is a physical organ in the body, it can be located and touched, and dissected. How about the mind? Is there a place it can be located? Surely there's no place in the body where it can be located. Now for many people, they use the brain and mind interchangeably to mean the same thing. But are they different from each other? Related to each? Does one control the other or does one emerge from the activities of the other? These are all philosophical, psychological, neurological, and medical questions that academics and expert professionals have been asking ever since the dawn of reason. And more than ever, the need for a more practical answer to these questions has never been so important as it is now. A better answer to the questions means better health, a healthier aging process, better mental health for diseased patients amongst many other things.

What we know at the moment is that the mind is a psychological process that only functions in conscious beings. If you have no brain or your brain is dead, you cannot be conscious and as a result, your mind can not produce thoughts. We also notice that the psychological minds of children are not fully functional until around the ages of 7 to 13 years. During this period, essential parts of the brain are not fully developed until around the same time. What this tells is that, not only is there a clear relationship between the brain and the mind, it seems the mind follows the processes of the brain in its maturation and operation. If your hippocampus is removed, you won't be able to remember any other thing that will happen after it has been removed. What seems to be the case is that the brain is the hardware that produces the software called the mind. If you tamper with the hardware, the software will equally be affected. And if the software can control the hardware in the same way you can shut down your laptop just by giving instructions to the software that runs it. The computer was modeled after the human neuropsychological architecture. And what studies from neuroscience, psychology, computer science, and neural networks tell us is that the health of your computer and your body are all dependent on the effective functioning of the software that runs them. The health of your body is dependent on the health of your mind. This is not a groundbreaking statement or discovery. There are billions and millions of articles, books, and videos that explain the phenomenon behind this much better than I have laid out here. But my intention here is to show you the role of communication, especially in the mind, in creating your health.

Communication as a means of expression is simply the communication of the internal processes of the mind which create the physical expressions that you perceive. From the way, you feel to speech production all depends on what is happening in your mind. Care, therefore, must be taken to handle what's happening in the mind for it is the wellspring of your life.

What we know at the moment is that when you think, the input from your mind activates the brain. The energy generated when we put our minds to work produces huge effects on our brain and causes our brains to organize our brain cells to instruct cells in our bodies to act in certain ways - usually as instructed.

The Role of the Heart in Communication.

Here is yet another organ in the body that plays an important role in the mind/body's relationship with communication. The heart.

The body of science known as Neurocardiology studies the role of the heart as an intelligent system in the neuropsychological functioning of an individual. Neurocardiology studies the interaction between the nervous system and the cardiovascular system. It describes stress-related cardiomyopathy, as exemplifying the brain-heart connection and how it arises in several conditions with acute brain injury and the same over-sympathetic response. A few broad categories summarize Neurocardiology: heart-brain relationships (e.g., cardiac source embolic stroke), brain-heart relationships (e.g., neurogenic heart disease), and neurocardiac syndromes (e.g., Friedreich disease).

What is the relationship between the heart, brain, and communication?

Toward the end of his distinguished career as Professor of Physiology at Harvard Medical School, Walter B. Cannon published a paper entitled "Voodoo Death," in which he recounted anecdotal experiences, largely from the anthropology literature of death from fright. A number of features characterized the events, which often came from remote places around the world. In these cases, all victims believed in absolute terms that the demise of the victim or themselves could be caused by an external supernatural force, such as a witch or medicine man, and that the victim could not alter this.

The victim's perceived inability to control a powerful external force is the sine qua non for all the cases recounted by Cannon, who postulated that death was caused "by a lasting and intense action of the sympathico-adrenal system."

According to Cannon, this phenomenon is limited to societies in which the people are "so superstitious, so ignorant, that they feel like strangers in a hostile land". In the absence of knowledge, they are susceptible to the power of an unrestrained imagination which inundates their surroundings with all manner of evil spirits capable of causing them great harm.

In essence, ill-health and death can be communicated to a person and the person will die. This can happen even without any physical intervention, but by just making them believe the words that have been spoken

Several decades have passed since Cannon made his observations, and evidence has built to support his hypothesis that "voodoo" death is, indeed, a real phenomenon but, far from being confined to ancient societies, it has the potential to reveal the biological basis for sudden death in contemporary societies and provide a window into the world of neurovisceral disease (also known as psychosomatic illness).

George Engel collected 160 accounts from the lay press of sudden deaths influenced by disruptive life events. He found that such events could be categorized into eight categories:

(a) The impact of death or collapse of a close person;

(2) During acute grief;

(3) Upon threat of loss of another close person;

(4) During mourning or an anniversary;

(5) On loss of status or confidence;

(6) Personal danger or threat of injury;

(7) After the danger is over;

(8) Reunion, triumph, or happy ending.

The common factor is that all of them involve events too important to ignore and in response to which victims are overwhelmed, give up, or both.

Curt Richter reported on a series of experiments aimed at elucidating Cannon's "voodoo" death. He incidentally discovered the rapid decline of rodent populations as a direct result of the sudden death of a colony of animals induced by the cutting off of the whiskers by Gordon Kennedy, a former classmate of Cannon in 1957. Richter studied the swimming time of domesticated rats in different water temperatures and found that the animals could swim for a maximum of 60 to 80 minutes at a temperature of 93°C. The animal, however, would drown within minutes if its whiskers were trimmed.

He noticed that the tendency for sudden death occurred for fierce wild rats as well, due to a number of factors including restraint, which involved enclosing them in a glass swimming jar with no chance of escape. Rats whose whiskers were trimmed, resulting in the destruction of the rats' most important proprioceptive mechanism, were at greater risk for early death. The presence of restraint and confinement was not a significant stressor for calm domesticated animals, however, the removal of whiskers induced fear in them as they were as fearful as wild rats, with the same tendency for death.

In addition, ECGs revealed bradycardia before death, suggesting that adrenalectomy didn't protect the animals. Moreover, atropine protected some of the animals, while cholinergic drugs led to a faster death. This led to the conclusion that increased vagal tone, not overactivity of the sympathetic nervous system, was responsible for the death.

In 1991, Dr. Armour discovered that the heart has a "little brain" or "intrinsic cardiac nervous system." This "heart brain" has nearly 40,000 neurons similar to brain neurons, meaning that the heart has its own nervous system. Also, the heart communicates with the brain in several ways: neurophysiologically, biochemically, biophysically, and energetically. 80% of the vagus nerve's connections are afferent, which means it sends information to the brain from the heart and other internal organs. The "heart brain" sends signals to the medulla, hypothalamus, thalamus, amygdala, and cerebral cortex. Therefore, the heart sends more signals to the brain than the brain sends to the heart. Pain perception has been shown, in studies, to be modulated by neural pathways and methods targeting the heart, such as vagus nerve stimulation and heart-rhythm coherence techniques. The heart does more than pump blood around the body. It has its own neural network, what we call its "little brain," and Methods that target the heart modulate brain regions dealing with pain.

The Relationship Between the Heart and The Brain

What does this mean for communication?

Communication between the heart and brain is key to understanding words and beliefs that create our state of health.

The cases of voodoo death show the relationship between thought-induced belief and state of health. In native Igbo eastern Nigeria where I am from, cases of voodoo death are a real thing. Growing up, there were many stories of a real victim of this kind of reality. There were even instances of voodoo sickness where people suffered from one sickness or the other just because of a belief that a wizard or witch doctor had placed a curse on them. Ailments like these ranged from simple causes like elephantiasis (a common occurrence to severe cases like heart disease, yes, heart!

On the other side, there are cases of placebo-induced healing that bring about - most times - the full restoration of severe health issues. These cases usually involve when a sick person

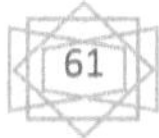

(probably an individual by voodoo belief) visits a church and his mindset is rejigged through the effective communication of new thoughts that shift their internal monologue. This usually leads to a full restoration of health. The mind communicates to the internal mechanisms of the body's cells, tissues, and organs. The right energy vibration restores them to full functionality.

Africans especially, the Igbo, have a very vibrant susceptible credulity that induces their belief. They can believe in voodoo death as much as they can believe in placebo. The only thing is that in most cases they don't have control over these beliefs and how they control their minds. This is because of an obvious absence of an uneducated internal monologue. The absence of this allows the thoughts planted by others to nurture and mature into full-blown beliefs that control one's life. Thus the overthink issues causing anxiety and heart palpitations that lead to general health breakdown.

Thoughts are the basis for your internal and external communication. Your communication creates your health; your health creates your life.

Managing your health begins with learning how to manage your thoughts. You do this by learning to control what you communicate within your internal monologue. This enables you to control what you profess to the world. Your words are a means of communicating your internal energy to the external world. You plant your thoughts in the world through verbal communication. You must take charge of your verbal communication. You don't take care of your verbal communication when you are about to pronounce the words, you take charge of it during your internal monologue. This is how health is created through communication.

Principles and Strategies for Thinking

Communication begins within before it is expressed outside. If you are going to take charge of your external communication, you must begin from within.

To do this there are principles and strategies you must apply to get you to take charge of your internal communication.

First, I begin with principles for effective internal communication. How to create the thinking and thoughts determine the language:

1. All thoughts are neutral until you interpret them. Your interpretation of thoughts gives the thought its quality - negative or positive.

2. Any thought you focus on magnifies. Every thought you could take over your cognitive space if you continually think about it. Your job is to train your mind to handle your thoughts so that only empowering thoughts occupy your cognitive space.

3. The quality of your mind determines the quality of your thoughts, the quality of your thoughts determines the quality of your life. You build the quality of your mind through study, reflection, meditation, metacognition, and hearing empowering messages often.

4. The quality of your thoughts determines the quality of energy in your body, the tone of your internal energy will determine the state of your health.

5. Thoughts are produced in the subconscious mind from where they are spread across the mind and control 95% of your life. Maintain mental vigilance to monitor the quality of thoughts that pop out from the subconscious now and again.

6. Every thought that saturates your subconscious mind drouks your cells with its equivalent energy.

7. Internal monologue is your access to your subconscious mind

8. An educated internal monologue produces an educated internal language.

9. Your internal language sets the default tone of how you will feel.

10. The predominant feeling you have is the signature tone of the quality of thought in your subconscious mind.

11. You can take charge of your internal monologue by practicing metacognition, meditation, and applying the rules of clear thinking.

12. The rules of clear thinking entail using intelligent questioning to access your thoughts before you engage them. Thinking from first principles instead of analogy, whenever you're confronted with any question or problem.

PART TWO –

COMMUNICATE

Communication is an art. It is an art that requires thoughtful execution and tact. It is an art that requires focus and attentiveness. To understand the art of communication, you must master the cognitive processes behind thought generation. For what is communicated is simply an expression of what is harbored in the mind. The essence of communication is to exercise influence and influence is a game of the mind not of mere words. Words will be barren and shallow if there is no articulated thought imbuing their essence. As an art, the communicator must become an artist by embodying the artistic virtues of tactful communication. To understand how to exercise this tact, you must understand the physics of communication. You must understand its makeup and deployment mechanism. Only when you have mastered this art can you exercise considerable influence over your interlocutor. Communication is a game. To play it, you must master it.

CHAPTER FOUR

THE OLD MAN, HIS THROAT AND THOUGHTS

Old age and sickness bring out the essential characteristics of a man". So says Felix Frankfurter. But was the same thing to be said of this man?

He was in his 70's when he developed a swallowing difficulty and decided to visit the hospital. Sam Londe was a retired shoe salesman who lived outside St. Louis during the early 1970s. He started having swallowing complications, when he visited a physician who discovered he was suffering

Metastatic Esophageal Cancer (cancer of the esophagus), a sickness still novel as at that time.

His doctor advised him to have surgery to get rid of the cancer which he agreed to. As things turned out, Londe's cancer, instead of receding, spread throughout his entire left lobe liver.

The subsequent news from his doctor was that he had just months to live.

Having heard such unfortunate news, Londe who had earlier lost his wife including all he's worked for his entire life in an earthen dam failure, became ever more devastated.

But as luck would have it, Londe met with another woman who cared for him, regardless of his loss and sickness. Shortly after the doctor declared him close to death, Londe and his wife decided to move over to Nashville where his wife's family stayed. Soon he was admitted to a nearby hospital while placed under the care of his new physician- Clifton Meador. The first time Meador set eyes on him, he felt concerned about his looks as he lay in a fetal position, looking debilitated and unforthcoming.

Londe was soon diagnosed with high blood glucose level as a result of diabetes, with a minimal higher level of liver enzymes, and every other test proved negative. With the aid of Dr. Meador Londe began therapy sessions accompanied by a fluid diet. Londe began to loosen his gloom while becoming more responsive. He shared his life story with Dr. Meador who was moved by what he heard and inquired what he could do to help his condition. "Just help me make it through Christmas", was Londe's response. Dr. Meador assured him he was going to do all within his powers.

In October, Londe was discharged, looking fit and proper to the amazement of everyone including Dr. Meador. But just a week after Christmas Londe was brought back to the hospital looking dying again. The x-ray performed on him showed a slight fever and a sign of pneumonia. The blood test run on him was all negative, and he was prescribed antibiotics, while placed under oxygen, but within 24hours, Sam Londe was dead.

An autopsy performed on him found very little cancer in his body, certainly not sufficient to kill him.

There were a couple of spots in the liver and one in the lung, but there was no trace of esophageal cancer that everyone thought had killed him!

Three decades later, Meador told the Discovery Health Channel: "He died with cancer, but not from cancer. "I thought he had cancer. He thought he had cancer. Everybody around him thought he had cancer. Did I remove hope in some way?"

Truly Thoughts are things and powerful things at that. So says Napoleon Hill

Communication - Expression - Verbal and Non-Verbal

I would like to begin this section of the book with interestingly pessimistic and humoristically formulated observations about human communication by Professor Osmo Antero Wiio in 1978.

It's known as Wiio's law. The law states that "Communication usually fails, except by accident". The full set of laws is as follows:

1. Communication usually fails, except by accident.

    a) If communication can fail, it will.

    b) If communication cannot fail, it still most usually fails.

    c) If communication seems to succeed in the intended way, there's a misunderstanding.

    d) If you are content with your message, communication certainly fails.

2.	If a message can be interpreted in several ways, it will be interpreted in a manner that maximizes the damage.

3.	There is always someone who knows better than what you meant with your message.

The more we communicate, the worse communication succeeds.

5. The more we communicate, the faster misunderstandings propagate. In mass communication, the important thing is not how things are but how they seem to be.

6.	The importance of a news item is inversely proportional to the square of the distance.

7.	The more important the situation is, the more probable you had forgotten an essential thing that you remembered a moment ago.

The whole point of this law is to let you know that as trivial as it might appear to you, communication is a serious business that cannot be taken for granted. It is a system that if left to its

own devices without proper thought and effort applied in its conduct, will result in utter degeneration. Therefore, effort must be taken to handle it with care and reason. Because lives depend on it.

The first step towards doing this is to gain an understanding of what communication is.

Communication is a form of expression. An expression of thought and ideas.

Language evolved as a means to help humans communicate their thoughts and ideas. Up until its evolution, like many other animals, humans struggled to communicate their thoughts, ideas, and feelings. This caused a lot of time lag between thought and execution. In interpreting the world that time difference meant a lot. It is the difference between survival and extinction in most cases. If you look at the history of species in the evolutionary time scale, you'll find that the ability of any species or life form to survive and pass on its genes successfully to the next generation, rests in its ability to organize its

intelligence effectively to get things done. This is largely achieved by reducing the lag time between thinking and execution. One of the best ways to organize intelligence is through collaboration. But you cannot collaborate with others if you can't communicate. And if you can communicate, your ability to survive depends strictly on how effectively and efficiently you can do it. Efficiency entails that it costs you less time and energy to communicate, while effectiveness means that you can communicate clearly, accurately and get tasks done. Efficiency and effectiveness is a determinant for successful communication. The species that scores highest on the ladder of efficiency and effectiveness can get to the top of the food chain.

It is believed by researchers that language probably evolved with consciousness. This is because the areas of the brain that account for conscious thought and execution - the prefrontal cortex - are also hugely implicated in the processing of language. What this means is that it could be that as we humans evolved consciousness, our level of intelligence was so sophisticated and high that it could not be contained only in one individual, therefore we needed to share it. The level of sophistication our conscious thoughts took on required sharing and collaboration for it to be effective, less it becomes destructive. This probably explains why when you lock up your thoughts and emotions within you for some time, you fall into depression. The level of energy that conscious thoughts and ideas carry is so much that a single mind cannot process it. There is a need to get a second mind to share the energy with and a third and a fourth. By doing so the energy becomes a creative force instead of a destructive one.

Language is an organized thought communicated through speech. Its effect in the world is determined by the level of organization and clarity that goes into its processing. We use language for verbal communication. As a tool of communication, language requires thought and clarity for it to achieve its goal.

Language as a means of communication is not strictly restricted to speech. Speech is the articulation of thought and production of verbal sound. Language on the other hand involves many types of communication including other forms of expression like sign language, facial expressions, gesticulations, even bodily movements. All of these have a way of communicating meaning to the other person.

The essence of language is to communicate thought in a meaningful form that your interlocutor can understand.

An interlocutor is the recipient of your message.

Meaning is organized and useful thought.

In Communicating meaning, care must be taken so that what is communicated is actually what is intended.

In the healthcare setting the ultimate goal in clinician-patient interaction is the communication of a meaningful message that would lead to health. In other words, the essence is to communicate health. I have explained in the first part of this book that communication starts first in the mind -

primarily the subconscious mind - before it is expressed externally in either speech or any other form of language. In the same way our primary means of communicating - language - is not restricted to verbal language. There are equally other means of using language that is non-verbal. What this means, therefore, is that as a healthcare provider, your job is to ensure that in whatever way you are communicating to the patient, that you send a message that communicates health. Your job is to understand other forms of language and when you use them unknowingly.

You cannot achieve this if your mind is not set to the default state that communicates health. To be effective in doing this as a healthcare practitioner, you must be healthy in the mind before you can communicate health. What we communicate essentially is "thought" nothing else. If your thoughts are healthy then your message will bear healthy energy that will bring about heath. On the other hand, if they are toxic, stressed, and anxious, then you can't help it. *Nemo dat quod non habet,* meaning " no one gives what they do not have".

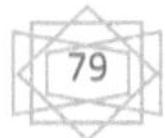

As I explained in part one, it is the task of every healthcare provider to put in enough work in rejigging their mindset. Now, the ultimate yardstick for measuring an effective healthcare provider is by measuring the quality of their mindset. The mindset is the place where health is first communicated before it is expressed. As a healthcare provider when you meet a patient what you do is simply an expression of "Who you are" and "What you are." Who you are is a product of your knowledge, "What you are" is a manifestation of your mindset (thought processes). The job you are performing at the moment is simply a manifestation of your learning and the state of your mind.

Most healthcare providers focus so much on "Who they are", - on their knowledge and training as a medical practitioner while neglecting "What they are" as healthcare providers - someone whose job is to communicate health.

Communicating health is an art that has to be learned. It is not automatically bequeathed to you on the day of graduation from medical or nursing school. It is a culture of the mind that has to be cultivated through conscious practice and eternal vigilance.

"What you are" determines your personality. As a healthcare provider, your job is to be a caregiver and not just an instructor. When you focus only on "who you are", you are focusing on the head knowledge of your practice. In that case, you are only an instructor. You're not focusing on the second part that plays an important role in communicating health to the patient. As a healthcare provider, you should have a balanced personality that incorporates professional knowledge and practical wisdom. The combination of both brings about a balanced healthcare provider that can communicate health to the patient - what I call a healthcare giver. More on this concept in part three.

Every healthcare provider should practice an exercise in clear thinking, as the learning coach Ugo Chukwu, admonishes in his book, "An exercise in clear thinking". A set of mental practices that enables you to process information accurately and fast enough. This is an important point because as a healthcare provider you are not inoculated from falling into the ditch of disempowering beliefs, biases, and prejudices that often inhibit you from thinking clearly and communicating health to the patient.

It is indeed a tragedy when a healthcare provider becomes prejudiced and biased over his patient.

This situation tantamount to catastrophe.

Your ability to communicate health rests solely on how you feel about the patient - interlocutor. When your beliefs lead you to start thinking about your patient from the lens of race, gender, ethnicity, and social class, then you lose the ability to make a sound judgment based on empirical data of science that is presented before you. In this case, there's no balance between "What you are" and "Who you are". You have allowed your poor beliefs to truncate your practical knowledge of medicine. This disharmonic proportion of energy within you will inevitably lead to one thing - poor communication that does nothing but harm to your patient.

An exercise in clear thinking helps you to create a mental framework that guides your judgment based on observed laws of nature rather than the prejudiced beliefs and opinions we have inherited from our culture and traditions. This will enable you to make balanced judgments based on knowledge and practical wisdom.

Communication begins in the mind before they are manifested in your external expressions. If you must manage communication to reflect the health and wellbeing you intend for your patient, then it begins with learning how to think clearly so that you can communicate clearly and effectively.

How to Think Clearly and Communicate Health

Evaluate your personality and psychological needs: we have a signature personality that is born out of a combination of factors, including our genetic predisposition and environmental conditioning.

There's an interesting theory in psychology that explains human behavior and trait qualities. It's called the Big 5 personality traits developed from the 1980s onwards in psychological trait theory. It serves as a measure to assess human trait qualities based on their natural inclinations and dispositions. The Big 5 personality traits are extraversion (also often spelled extroversion), agreeableness, openness, conscientiousness, and neuroticism.

Each trait represents a continuum. Individuals can fall anywhere on the continuum for each trait. The Big 5 remains relatively stable throughout most of one's lifetime. They are influenced significantly by both genes and the environment, with an estimated heritability of 50%. They are also known to predict certain important life outcomes such as education and health.

An understanding of these big 5 traits plays a pivotal role in thinking and communicating effectively. The big 5 traits determine to a large extent how you are going to react or respond to a certain situation. For someone who is high in neuroticism, their communication pattern will be different from a person who is low in neuroticism and high in openness, people who are high in neuroticism are easily irritable and conservative. This might affect their communication pattern as they tend to be less open to conversations and are easily provoked by even seemingly harmless offhand comments. They hold grudges and suffer from them. We see this in the angry patients who tend to be rude to their clinicians.

Those who are high in agreeableness tend to be less assertive. Those who are high in extroversion tend to fall into the category of talkative and sometimes inpatient patients. Those who are high in openness tend to be the inpatient patient and sometimes too assertive. While those who are high on conscientiousness tend to be sometimes the knowledgeable patient who questions the knowledge of the clinician, especially

when they suspect any sign of lack of confidence. They sometimes tend to be the patient who follows the clinician's instructions and meets up with doctor's appointments.

As a clinician, a basic understanding of psychology will serve you well in interfacing with your patients. You are interacting with humans, therefore, you must understand how they think and behave before you can actually help them. Healthcare is a holistic system that involves all aspects of human wellbeing including psychology, biology as well as physiology.

An understanding of human personality traits enables you to interface with your patients better. But more importantly, it allows you to do something much more - understanding yourself so that you can serve others from a place of strength rather than a place of weakness.

An understanding of the big 5 traits enables you to make a clear assessment of your psychological and temperamental dispositions. This will give you an analytic graph of who you are, allowing you to know how to react to almost any situation you find yourself in.

The graph of who you are - your personality - enables you to practice metacognition. To monitor and catch your thoughts before they are expressed. It allows you to educate your internal monologue so that you can exercise control over your dominating thoughts. It enables you to monitor your beliefs and know how they affect your life.

When you understand yourself and understand others within the spectrum of these big 5 traits. It allows you to practice emotional dexterity - the ability to monitor your exact emotions and your environment to access them for the appropriate response.

Self-Awareness is key to communicating better. You understand yourself first before you understand others. As Osinakachi Akuma Kalu said, "don't waste your time trying to understand others when you have not yet understood yourself."

The process of applying these principles of clear thinking is therefore to first try and understand yourself within the spectrum of the big 5 traits, then try to understand how others equally fit within this spectrum.

You might ask yourself but how do I accurately assess my patient's psychological disposition when I just met him or her? This is a very important and valid question to ask. The good news is that it doesn't require a lot of expertise. It only requires common sense.

Whenever you encounter a patient during your consultation try and assess their personality by asking them basic questions about their interests, family, close relationships, and work. Ask them about their day. Look out for fillers of personality traits in their answers. Whether they love hanging out or studying indoors, whether they are passionate to achieve new milestones, lead their team or they prefer to follow the lead of other competent leaders. Their answers to your unsuspecting questions will give you a window into the soul of their personality.

A good understanding of the big 5 traits will set you up to understand the second criteria and deploy it in your work.

Evaluate your beliefs: This is key to thinking clearly and making judgments.

People's values say a lot about their past and personality.

But from where do values emerge? What do we think about them? And how do we set them?

Every human action begins with a thought that is organized in the form of an idea. When an idea hijacks our biological system and sets in place the release of neurotransmitters that produce hormones that control the emotional centers of our brain, it produces a belief. Beliefs are memories, they are encoded feelings in our minds and bodies. Beliefs are developed as stimuli received as trusted information and stored in the memory. These perceptions are generalized and

established into beliefs. They have their own intelligence that can cause us to act even when we are unwilling.

Our values begin with our beliefs.

Beliefs can be a very powerful mechanism for creating our lives. They play an important role in who we are and in determining what we hold dear most.

Beliefs are very powerful tools for creating and acting in the world. Understood from a psychological perspective, belief is the feeling of certainty that makes you accept something as true. From a biological perspective, belief is simply the release of the neurotransmitter dopamine that is produced in the substantia nigra, ventral tegmental area, and hypothalamus of the brain. When this hormone is released, it produces a feeling of certainty that makes the person accept whatever is presented as true and thus motivated to act in accordance.

In order to stabilize belief and respond to the environment, whole-brain function is needed. Brain regions and neural circuits play an important role in establishing beliefs and executing emotions. The frontal lobe plays a major role in beliefs. Mental representations of the world are integrated with sub-cortical information by the prefrontal cortex. Amygdala and Hippocampus are involved in the process of thinking and thus assist in the execution of beliefs. Thinking and beliefs are influenced by the N-methyl-D-aspartate receptor (NMDA). It is possible to challenge these beliefs. As a belief is challenged more, it becomes stronger. A new stimulus creates distress in the brain when it is combined with existing patterns. The distress triggers the release of dopamine (neurotransmitter) to transmit the signal.

Liane Young, a Professor of Psychology, at Boston College and Rebecca Saxe a Professor of Cognitive Neuroscience, at MIT in their 2008 paper *The neural basis of belief encoding and integration in moral judgment.* found that the medial prefrontal cortex is involved in processing belief valence. The right temporoparietal junction and precuneus are involved in the processing of beliefs into moral judgment.

The right temporoparietal junction is responsible for processing true beliefs. Using examples from children's judging of belief questions on short stories, Saxe explains that beliefs judgment begins at the age of five. The regions of the medial prefrontal cortex, the superior temporal gyrus, and the hippocampal area are activated during belief attribution. Researchers have found that dopamine levels are associated with paranormal thoughts, suggesting that dopamine plays a role in belief development.

A Belief in itself is neither true nor false, it's simply a feeling of certainty. This feeling can be inspired by a form of knowledge. The knowledge motivating it could be real or imagined, true or false, fact or fantasy. It only needs to be convincing enough to activate the certain centers of your brain to release the necessary hormones to get you to act.

Beliefs are very important because, without them, we cannot get ourselves to act on anything. We need belief to act on everything. From buying snacks to getting a degree. From playing a game to crossing a street with a traffic light. Our cells even need belief most. Without belief, our cells cannot carry out the most basic metabolic processes in our system. We can't perform basic physiological and bodily functions. We can't heal, most importantly we cannot be healthy. Explaining how this works, Sathyanarayana Rao T.S. and his colleagues in their paper on *"The biochemistry of belief,"* Explains that:

> The biochemistry of our body stems from our awareness. Belief-reinforced awareness becomes our biochemistry. Each and every tiny cell in our body is perfectly and absolutely aware of our thoughts, feelings and of course, our beliefs. There is a beautiful saying 'Nobody grows old. When people stop growing, they become old'. If you believe you are fragile, the biochemistry of your body unquestionably obeys and manifests it. If you believe you are tough (irrespective of your weight and bone density!), your body undeniably mirrors it. When you believe you are depressed (more precisely, when you become consciously aware of your 'Being depressed'), you stamp the raw data received through your sense organs, with a judgment — that is your personal view

– and physically become the 'interpretation' as you internalize it. A classic example is 'Psychosocial dwarfism', wherein children who feel and believe that they are unloved, translate the perceived lack of love into depleted levels of growth hormone, in contrast to the strongly held view that growth hormone is released according to a preprogrammed schedule coded into the individual's genes! ...Thoughts and beliefs are an integral part of the brain's operations. Neurotransmitters could be termed the 'words' brain uses to communicate with exchange of information occurring constantly, mediated by these molecular messengers. Unraveling the mystery of this molecular music induced by the magic of beliefs, dramatically influencing the biochemistry of the brain could be an exciting adventure and a worth pursuing cerebral challenge.

Belief acts as one of the most powerful stimulants of life.

Its power is so much that it could act as a double-edged sword.

It helps life to function smoothly. At the same time, it could

destroy life if applied wrongly.

We usually use the concept of belief in religious settings thinking its mention and application can only be within the spaces of religious circles. But belief is equally relevant in the healthcare system, if not even more important.

Oftentimes we misunderstand the healthcare space as just strictly a science-fact-based setting. While this should be true, unfortunately, and fortunately it's not. The reason is simple: we humans are belief-centered beings. We can't operate only in the realm of facts. Our psychology did not evolve to do that alone. When we are only science and fact-based we lose touch with our emotions and empathy. It is belief that allows us to feel and care, nurture and encourage. Belief in itself is not only a psychological reality, it's equally a biological one. Hence the importance of understanding how it functions and is applied in the healthcare setting.

The entire healthcare sector has been set firmly on a foundation of a belief system. People trust scientific facts because they believe in their assumptions, theories, and facts.

The scientific process has from the time of Aristotle to the time of Francis Bacon been tested and proven to be a solid process for ascertaining truth. From the time of Bacon to now, its truth value has only been further cemented to the point that in places like the west and America, science has become like the word of God - unquestionable and indubitable. We, therefore, take the words of scientists as holy and ex-cathedra, even when their opinions are not yet conclusive on a subject matter. We have successfully created a scientific belief system. One that upholds the theories and method of its process as the ultimate truths of life.

The healthcare sector is part of this belief-based science community. This belief system has been successfully communicated to the general public. This is where the trust we have in our healthcare system comes from. You trust that when you go to the hospital whatever the clinician tells you is at least 95% true. And if you're like most people it's 100% true. Your belief comes from centuries of questioning of this system and its validation through its process. After centuries of testing, it

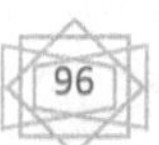

has proved and continues to prove itself through our technologies, which medicine is one of them.

The placebo effect is a phenomenon that has shown that people can become healed whole and hearty just from the belief they express over the medicine and what they have been told about it. Some estimates have it that the majority of the healing that occurs in the healthcare system is attributable to a placebo. If estimates like these are anything close to the truth even by a fraction, what it means is that belief is an indispensable tool in the sector, therefore as a healthcare provider, you should understand it and deploy it in your medical process.

Values come from beliefs: Values are a set of principles that control one's actions based on their beliefs.

It is a crucial aspect of thinking clearly and communicating well with your patient. To become an effective health care provider, you must learn to access your value system and that of your patient to understand what their needs and priorities are in life. This is part of the effective process of understanding the psychology of your patient.

When you understand the psychology of your patient you understand their needs, wants, hopes, aspirations, dreams, visions, and goals. These are the things that run their lives. This is why they wake in the morning to do what they do. You cannot effectively manage their biology if you don't understand their psychology. To a large extent, psychology conditions biology. And vice versa. Values are the psychological needs of people that determine their modus operandi.

When you understand the value system of your patient you understand why they talk and behave the way they do. It even gives you a clue as to their type of personality trait. This allows you to access the kind of attention to give to them and in what ways.

The problem now becomes how do you determine one's value system, when you barely have enough time to spend with the patient? To solve that you have to understand that values are portrayed from both verbal and nonverbal clues.

Understand what they say: You get information about the value system of your patient through verbal cues like the kind of words and phrases they use most often.

The quality of their language whether positive or negative? The tone of their voice is soft or harsh. What they profess faith in and how they do it. For example, statements like I believe my family and I are destined for greatness if we work at it, irrespective of the conditions in the country.

What they profess hope for. I just wish for the day this illness goes away so that I can enjoy a great time with my family.

These cues in their language say a lot about their personality hidden away from the facade of their common expression.

Nonverbal expressions: Nonverbal expressions are even more important because they act as the window to the soul of our personality. Verbal expression is a rational process. Because language evolved with rational thinking, it is often subjected to the scrutiny of reason. Through this means our thoughts are often edited before they are produced. Our verbal expressions, therefore, do not bear the full weight of our thoughts and intentions within, in short, they don't express the purity of our personality.

But with nonverbal expressions, there is a greater chance of peering into the soul of a person if you understand how they work. Take for instance facial expressions. They say a lot about how we feel from moment to moment. From a grimace to a smile, there is a huge amount of information that is locked away behind each muscle movement on the face. The reason for this is simple. Most times even when we think we are, we can't control the muscle contractions on our face or our body movements. These reactions usually come before words are articulated. The reason is that these muscles on the face and other parts of the body are connected to the autonomic nervous system which controls involuntary movements.

Our facial expressions can either be honest (based on the way we feel) or forced (based on what we want to express, even though we feel differently.) The emotional center (limbic system) and the volitional center (motor cortex) are located in two different parts of the brain.

Our limbic system is known as our "factory of emotions". The system works the same way in animals and humans alike.

When we feel an emotion, it is immediately reflected in our facial expression, or our body language, or most often, in both. In humans, it is the same formation that has evolved over many eons. Just by looking at someone's face, we can unmistakably recognize joy or surprise, curiosity or anxiety, anger or disgust, regardless of their race or gender.

The limbic system is capable of making facial muscles highly specific and highly differentiated, largely due to our experience of (and need to express) a wide range of emotions.

The motor cortex controls facial movements in a much coarser and less nuanced manner than the limbic system. We can usually tell a genuine smile from a fake one, and a genuine surprise from a staged one. Subconsciously, we notice the difference.

When we express ourselves with a facial expression, whether it is a spontaneous emotional reaction or a planned expression, our brain sends signals to the facial nerve from the limbic system and the motor cortex. The nucleus of the facial nerve combines the signals arriving from both centers, and our face reflects the results.

The limbic system is part of the central nervous system, which includes your brain and spinal cord. More specifically, the limbic system is a set of brain structures that includes the hippocampus and amygdala, and some others.

Human (actually, mammalian) physiology is characterized by the central nervous system as well as the somatic nervous system and autonomic nervous system.

The limbic system contains neurochemicals such as dopamine, noradrenaline, and serotonin. Pulse, blood pressure, respiratory rate, and arousal are all regulated by the autonomic nervous system and hypothalamus in response to emotional cues.

So when there's an internal communication of energy, the face, body, and eye automatically adjust with the internal mechanisms. Even without you being aware of these changes most of the time. Take for example the pupil of the eyes, they bear within them a vast amount of information about what is going inside our heads at every moment. Ancient philosophers and thinkers long before the science and technology to measure its role have hinted at its importance. Charlotte Bronte in the 1800s said, ``The soul, fortunately, has an interpreter - often an unconscious, but still a truthful interpreter - in the eye.''

With the aid of modern technology and science, we now know from research that the eye plays a link to the brain. For example, Duke University researchers have examined monkeys' eyes to gain insight into how the brain processes distractions and found that changes in pupil size in response to distractors predict how well the brain focuses.

Pupillometry is the study and measurement of pupil diameter and how it reacts to environmental stimuli and mental processes. It measures changes in pupil size in response to various types of stimulation to study pupillary responses. Additionally, pupillometry has revealed a top-down correlation between pupillary responses and some highly complex mental operations The process of top-down information processing involves information being sent from the brain to the body on a higher level. Specifically, perception, emotional responses, and cognitive load, the amount of mental effort used during information processing.

Pupillary activity is also known to be induced by brain structures, involved in higher-level activities, such as emotion and cognition (thinking). The regions of the brain that help us

feel emotions can also cause pupil dilation. Our environment can trigger emotional responses, either positive or negative, which can result in pupillary dilation. In one study, Partala and Surakka presented participants with a series of sounds and monitored their pupils as they listened. Participants scored the sounds as either positive, negative, or neutral at the end of each presentation. People with positive or negative opinions of a sound (such as a baby laughing) or a sound (such as a couple fighting), experienced greater pupil dilation as compared to people with neutral opinions (such as background office noises), which tended to have little effect on pupil size.

Daniel Kahneman, in his book, "Thinking Fast and Slow", talks about the role of the eye as the window to the soul. The movement of the pupil acts as a powerful tool for deciphering what is going on in the brain. It appears that the pupil dilates and expands based on the surge of energy that is going in the head. In research, they conducted at the University of Michigan. They found that participants when given a hard cognitive task to do, their pupils dilated as they thought about sometimes answers to the questions they were asked. As they kept thinking about the problem the pupil stays contracted, then when they suddenly figured it out, it expanded out again. It is as if the eye was showing the energy consumption level of the brain and the cognitive time it took them to process the question and come up with an answer.

By monitoring the activity and movement of the eye, you can understand when you ask someone a question, the weight and impact of that question on their brain. And by observing their involuntary facial muscle movements you can see through them to understand beyond what they are saying but what they are thinking.

CHAPTER FIVE

THE NATURE OF COMMUNICATION

In this chapter I'll help you understand the models, types, and levels of communication so that you can better appreciate how to apply the principles and lessons I have laid out in this book more practically in your work as a healthcare provider. If you're not a healthcare provider don't worry the ideas in this chapter will equally help you as the message has been addressed to all and sundry who genuinely wish to improve their communication skills.

We start here with interesting ideas from the ancient Greek philosopher Plato.

To explain his principles to his readers, Plato wrote dialogues.

Between 428 BC and 347 BC, Plato lived in Athens and was a distinguished Greek philosopher. Historically, his doctrine is considered to be of central importance to the foundation of Western culture.

As a philosopher, Plato authored numerous works, including dialogues in which the protagonist, generally the philosopher Socrates, interacts with various characters to discuss philosophical issues. These dialogues are intended to teach the student, who can learn valuable teachings by reading - or, even better, by listening to them. But above all, his dialogues lay out the rules of effective communication as I will share with you here.

Plato's Rules for Effective Communication

The first rule deals with knowledge of what one wants to communicate — the truth of the subject matter. You must think clearly about what you have in mind. To do this, take care to understand the ramifications and stakes of what is involved in what you intend to communicate. Plato advises that you must communicate the truth of the subject matter. This involves knowing the truth about what you want to communicate and communicating that truth without prevarication.

The second rule has to do with the psychology of the interlocutor/audience/listener: In communicating with your patient, who in this case is your interlocutor you must ensure that you understand their state of mind, level of education, belief systems, and personality traits. Only when you do this can you begin to appreciate the uniqueness of their peculiar circumstances and begin to apply it in your communication with them. More on the psychology of the patient is treated in the third part of this book.

The third rule deals with the reciprocal relationship of all parts of the communication— this means that good communication must be systematized and communicated like a living creature, where every part is harmoniously linked to another. This is at the heart of the democratic model of communication where the model is participatory instead of linear or dyadic.

The fourth rule speaks about the complementary procedure of communication which is synthesis— a good communication must be able to synthesize the different elements involved in communication. When interacting with a patient, approach their issue with a system thinking approach. Understand that nothing is to be left out in all that they have said. Everything mentioned in their report is important. They give viable information that can be utilized in proffering solutions. Synthesize all aspects of the communication, all data you have about the patient. Don't leave anything to chance because you can find that what you're looking for can come from the unlikeliest sources or you can find it in the combination of all sources.

To understand how to apply these, let's take a look at four models of communication to understand which model is the most useful in our communication.

An understanding of these models will enable you to know which one you are applying in any situation. If you understand which model of communication you are applying, then you will know how effective it will be, based on the peculiarity of your situation.

Linear Communication

The linear communication model explains the process of one-way communication, whereby a sender transmits a message and a receiver absorbs it. In this form, the message is transmitted to the receiver and decodes before he receives it.

Here the responsibility of decoding and understanding rests not on the sender but the receiver. Based on the nature of this model, many things can affect the one-way communication process. This one-way model of communication doesn't support effective feedback.

Dyadic Communication

In general, 'Dyadic communication' refers to an interaction between two individuals. Even if more than two persons are present in a situation, it is only two communicators that play a fundamental role. It is a person-to-person transaction and one of the commonest forms of speech communication.

Democratic Communication

A democratic model of communication uses a participatory model.

Based on the ideals of western liberal democracy, this form of communication promotes the equal participation of all involved in the communication process. Here the healthcare provider is expected to allow a mutual communicative framework. This model allows the patient to see the process of securing their health as one that is participatory where all efforts are directed towards helping them get better.

The democratic model offers the best model of communication in the healthcare setting. Because it allows the patient to participate in the healthcare process. It builds a strong relationship between the patient and the healthcare provider. It equally ensures effective cross-communication amongst all healthcare providers within the healthcare setting.

Plato's rule for effective communication serves as the best way to understand and apply the democratic model of communication.

CHAPTER SIX

TYPES OF COMMUNICATION

Verbal Communication:

When we speak to others, we engage in verbal communication. It can be face-to-face, over the phone, via Skype or Zoom, etc. Verbal engagements can be informal, such as chatting with a friend over coffee or in the office kitchen, or more formal, such as a scheduled meeting. Although words are important, it is equally important how we string those words together to convey an overall message as well as our intonation (pitch, tone, cadence, etc.) while speaking. While words are important when face-to-face, they cannot be separated from non-verbal communication.

The following are a few steps you can follow to improve your verbal communication skills:

- Your speaking voice should be strong and confident. Especially when presenting information to a patient, be sure to use a strong voice so that he or she can hear you easily. It is important to speak clearly and be easy for others to understand so that you will be understood.

- Keep filler words to a minimum. Especially during a presentation, it can be tempting to use filler words, such as "um," "like," "so" or "yeah." While this may feel natural after completing a sentence or pausing to collect your thoughts, it can also distract your patient. Consider taking a deep breath instead of using them when tempted.

The way we act while we speak often says more than the words themselves. Communication through non-verbal means includes facial expressions, posture, eye contact, hand movements, and touch. If you're speaking with your patient about health matters, for example, it is important to pay attention to both their words and non-verbal communication. Verbally, your patient might agree with your idea, but nonverbal cues such as avoiding eye contact, sighing, or scrunching up their faces suggest otherwise.

Develop your nonverbal communication skills by following these steps:

- Be aware of how you feel physically when you are feeling emotions. You will experience a range of emotions throughout the day (such as feeling energized, bored, happy or frustrated). Try to identify where in your body you feel that emotion. When you feel anxious, you might notice that your stomach feels tight. By becoming conscious of how your emotions impact your body, you can gain greater control over what you present externally. Your nonverbal communication grows from the inside to the outside.

- You should be intentional about your non-verbal communication. You should aim to display positive body language when you are alert, open, and optimistic about your surroundings. If you feel confused or anxious about information, you can also use body language to support your verbal communication, such as furrowing your brow. When asking follow-up questions or giving feedback, use body language as well as verbal communication.

- Try to mimic your favorite nonverbal communication style. You can use the facial expressions or body language you find beneficial in a certain setting as a guide when improving your own nonverbal communication. If you see that confirmation and approval are communicated efficiently by nodding your head, use it the next time you have the same feelings.

Written Communication

Regardless of the form of written communication - an email, a memo, a report, an article, a tweet, a contract - all of them share one purpose: to disseminate information concisely and clearly. However, this objective is rarely met. Poor writing skills can result in confusion and embarrassment, as well as legal problems. The most important aspect of written communication, especially in the digital age, is that the message lives on, perhaps forever. Thus, two points need to be kept in mind: First, write well, because poorly constructed sentences will make you appear incompetent. The second thing to do is to ensure the message is one you want to promote or be associated with long-term. As a healthcare provider, care must be taken with how you use social media channels, especially when it comes to sharing your opinions on health matters. You don't want to divulge patient health-sensitive data in a public forum like Facebook or Twitter no matter how sincere your intentions are.

Listening

Listening does not often appear on the list of forms of communication. Active listening is perhaps one of the most important types of communication. This is because, if we do not listen to the person sitting right beside us, we cannot effectively interact with them.

Imagine a negotiation - a key step is to find out what the opposition demands. Without listening, it is impossible to assess this, which makes it difficult to achieve a win-win outcome. The same is true in a healthcare setting. As a clinician and more importantly, a healthcare giver, you must develop the art of active listening. See your communication with the patient as a form of negotiation. You're negotiating with the patient to conform to a new habit so that he can live healthily; you're

negotiating with the patient to take your advice and adhere to clinical prescriptions. All of these requests are equally difficult to adhere to. This is why communicating with the patient who finds himself in a situation where they are asked to "change" their old self and embrace a new version is not an easy task. It requires tactful communication.

Visual Communication

Visual culture is part of our daily lives. The TV runs 24/7, Facebook is visual with videos, memes, images, etc., Instagram is an image-only platform, advertisers use imagery to sell products and ideas. Take a moment to think about your social media posts from a personal perspective. They are meant to elicit emotion - to convey a message. Occasionally, the message will be to show off your accomplishments, for example, I just won an award or I am now a father Many of these displays are crafted to stir the hearts of viewers, particularly shots of injured animals or children in tears.

The entire day is filled with constant communication. We operate on automatic pilot when it comes to communication. However, I encourage you to consider how you communicate. What is your verbal communication style? When you are disinterested, what are your nonverbal cues? Are you excited? Do you feel Nervous? How well do you listen? How well can you write a concise, well-articulated message? How well do you communicate with others? Are there any barriers?

The first step to communicating more effectively is understanding how you communicate. Communication courses are easy to find online. A variety of credit and non-credit courses are available to help you improve your communication skills. I have developed a communication course drawn from my 30 thirty-year experience in communicating with patients in the healthcare setting. Check it out. If you find it helpful you can subscribe. If not, there are many others out there you can learn from.

Other Ways to Ensure Effective Visual Communication:

These steps are very helpful for clinicians who have an active social media presence.

- Before incorporating visuals, ask for feedback. Consider asking for feedback when sharing a visual aid in a presentation or email. Visuals can sometimes make a presentation more engaging, confusing, or muddled. You can decide whether a visual adds value to your communication by getting a third-party perspective.

-

- Think about your audience. Include visuals that are easily understood by your audience. If you are displaying a health chart with unfamiliar data, explain what is happening and how it relates to what you are saying. Never use sensitive, offensive, violent, or graphic visuals.

-

- Set personal goals to accomplish the things you want to accomplish step-by-step to improve your communication skills. Identify which areas would be best to focus on first with the help of trusted colleagues, managers, or mentors.

Communicating with Trust and Effectiveness

Storytelling

Storytelling is one of the most effective forms of verbal communication; it supports the formation of common meanings within healthcare settings by helping with communication. In organizations, stories can help clarify key values and demonstrate how things are done, and story frequency, strength, and tone are related to a higher level of

organizational commitment. This is no different in a healthcare setting. A clinician's ability to establish an effective relationship with the patient is related to the quality of the stories they tell. Stories can reinforce and perpetuate a culture in a patient. In the same way, it can help to build a relationship based on trust between the clinician and patient. When communicating a serious issue to a patient, that might demand a behavioral change or deliver a traumatic message like the death of a loved one. Stories go a long way in helping the patient or interlocutor absorb the emotional pressure that comes with the message. Stories bring us to a point of neutral assessment which allows us to process a message with minimal bias.

Conversations that matter

The process may be the same, but high-stakes communications require more planning, reflection, and skill than normal day-to-day interactions at work. Examples of high-stakes communication events include communicating the news of a terminal health issue or the news of the loss of a loved one. Apart from these occasions, there are many times in our professional lives when we have crucial conversations; conversations in which stakes are high, opinions differ, and emotions run high. Under these circumstances, the most consistent recommendation from communication experts is to use "and" rather than "but". You should also be aware of your communication style and be flexible; during stressful times, communication styles can become quite rigid. When to cut in and interrupt, when to maintain eye contact or look away to allow the other person to develop their train of thought, how you use gestures and body contact, the right tone to use depending on the nature of the message you're passing across. Your style of communication is as important as what you are communicating.

Written Communication

Health reports, prescriptions, memos, proposals, e-mails, letters, training manuals, operating policies, and books are all examples of written communications. You can print them out, write them by hand, or see them on a screen. Verbal communication normally takes place in real-time. Comparatively, written communication is constructed over time. It is common for written communication to occur asynchronously (at different times). A Sender can write a message that the receiver can read at any time, unlike a real-time conversation. Additionally, written communication can also be read by numerous people (e.g., all clinicians in a facility or all patients). It's a one-to-many situation communication, as opposed to a one-to-one verbal conversation. Of course, there are exceptions: a voicemail is an oral message that is asynchronous. Conference calls and speeches are one-to-many communications, while e-mails can be sent to only one recipient or many.

As a clinician or a patient, understand that just as there are many types of communication, so too are different styles and ways for communicating based on the style you have chosen. Your style of communication when you're using verbal communication cannot be the same when you are using communicating through writing. The mode of communication influences the style of communication. However, some things are central in the process. The tone of the message should be communicated across to engender the right attitude that you intend to communicate. The core of your message should be protected from the peculiar limitations of your type of communication. If you're texting a patient about the need to complete their dosage, it is not the same as when you call them on phone or conduct a video call, or talk of more when you talk to them face to face. All of these types of communication carry the same message with different energies. You must understand which type of communication will best deliver the core of your message.,

CHAPTER SEVEN

LEVELS OF COMMUNICATION

The first step to understanding different levels of communication is to understand what communication is. Every day, people communicate with each other. (with rare exceptions). Verbal communication occurs when we speak. We also communicate nonverbally, such as through body language, gestures, and demeanor. Our behavior also communicates. When we fail to follow through on our promises, it communicates something about our attitude and reliability.

It is astonishing to think that experts in the field have studied communication to the point of creating mathematical equations which represent the process of sending and receiving messages between individuals. Fortunately, the skills needed for understanding different levels of communication are not too complex. And you don't need to master the math. There is, however, one thing that one must understand: whichever way one communicates, how one communicates affects whether the interlocutor will be able to understand what the communicator intended to convey.

Different fields of study and different types of organizations classify levels of communication differently. Since communication occurs in innumerable ways, among billions of people every day in a wide range of circumstances, these classifications will always be somewhat arbitrary, because no single theory can explain every communication occurrence.

However, the classical view of communication generally involves four levels: intrapersonal, interpersonal, group, or communal. The best way to learn about these levels is to look at examples of each.

Intrapersonal Communication

Thinking is the most common form of intrapersonal communication.

Thinking, making notes to remind yourself what needs to be done, and talking to yourself are all examples of intrapersonal communication. At this level of communication, you are both the person sending and receiving the message. A powerful example of this mode of communication is the internal monologue which I mentioned in part one. You play these two roles so there are practically no opportunities for misinterpretation or miscommunication. But there could be a lack of clarity in your communication which could affect your interpersonal communication with others. You must understand that as a level of communication, it comes first before other levels. Thus, the first level of communication is where you begin learning to communicate before moving on to other levels. If you get it wrong on this level, you will most certainly get it wrong at other levels. Communication is first intrapersonal before it is interpersonal or communal.

Interpersonal Communication

Interpersonal communication includes talking to another individual, exchanging messages or emails, video conferencing, and even nonverbal means like shrugging one's shoulders. To consider interpersonal communication successful, the recipient must be able to understand the message that the sender intended to convey.

As an example, let's look at Emeka and Joyce. Let's go a little bit away from the clinical setting and to business. They are both members of the same marketing project team. Meetings are typically held with the rest of the marketing team, as well as representatives from the IT, human resources, and public relations departments who are contributing to the project. As can be seen in cross-departmental teams, participants from secondary teams have strong opinions about how something should be accomplished. For their meetings to proceed according to the agenda without interruptions from the IT representative, Emeka and Joyce need to be in sync. When the discussion starts to wander off course, they must be able to communicate clearly and quickly with one another, sometimes with just eye contact or a raised eyebrow. Through effective interpersonal communication, they can become more effective at their jobs.

When we say this person understands me very well. It is another way of saying my interpersonal communication with the person is highly effective and smooth. When someone understands you they understand almost all the way you communicate and they can use empathy to mirror your world. This is the highest form of interpersonal communication. When you use empathy to mirror other people's world, you go from listening and responding to what they are saying in words to embodying their ideas and feelings. You can perceive their energy and respond by hearing anything from them. This is the highest level of interpersonal communication.

Group or communal communication

Using Emeka, Joyce, and their team as an example, the activity they engage in every time they have a team meeting is an exercise in group communication. For group communication to be successful, every member of the group must be present, aware, and attentive to the messages being sent and received. Often, groups of this type require documents, such as meeting notes, agendas, and presentations, to ensure everyone agrees. Group communication demands a different set of skills than interpersonal communication since one sender must send a message to several receivers at the same time.

This is the sort of communication that can be witnessed in a hospital setting where there is a cross-communication relationship between different players in the healthcare system. Like between the doctors, nurses, patients, etc. Understanding

how to handle communication on a group level is key to building a conducive environment for work.

These first three are the major levels of communication, other levels of communication that could be useful to you are:

Auditory Level of Communication

Our voice, including our tone, range, volume, and speed, affects how others hear and interpret our messages. If you are talking to an introverted, thoughtful person, it will be beneficial for fast talkers to slow down their speech. In addition, how we pronounce, inflect, and place emphasis on certain words can affect how others interpret what we say. Communication on the auditory level can be accomplished by becoming aware of various auditory cues and speaking to others in a way that resembles their own (similar to "matching and mirroring").

Emotional Level of Communication

Only a few people are aware of how our emotional states affect what we communicate and how the message is interpreted. In rhetoric, Aristotle's pathos refers to the appeal to the audience's emotions. How much do you like people who are positive and life-affirming versus those who are negative and critical of others? Are you enthusiastic or boring? Speaker's emotions influence the recipient's state of mind and how the listener interprets what is said. To communicate effectively on an emotional level, become aware of your emotional state, learning to pause and release negative emotions before communicating with others. When delivered with pride, anger, or fear, your words are unlikely to meet with a positive reception.

Energetic Level of Communication

Also called the psychic level, this level of communication encompasses a vast range of unseen factors including a person's level of consciousness, the frequency or harmonics of the message, and other subtle energies.

Some people seem to have an "X-factor"—a unique presence—that naturally imparts their messages to others with greater receptivity and understanding. This is sometimes called "Reality Distortion Field". An effective influence great people like Steve Jobs, Bill Clinton, and Augustus Caesar had that enabled them to bend the will of many to theirs. Even in circumstances that seemed impossible and improbable.

To communicate more effectively, hold the highest intention for the other person's wellbeing. This requires a unique level of mindfulness generally cultivated through compassion practices. When we are centered in a state of mastery, we're more likely to access this psychic dimension that holds great treasures of insights into others, helping us communicate with greater ease.

Bringing all the Levels of Communication Together

Content is what we say; it's also the way we say. We communicate a message on the physical, auditory, emotional, and energetic levels. All levels of communication are interdependent, as they affect each other. Our body language is influenced by our emotional state, and our overall field impacts our state of mind. Understanding these various levels can be useful. We can become more patient in our speech and more compassionate towards others and ourselves when we realize the complexities inherent in human communication.

As healthcare givers, our work is delicate and vocational. We should assume the responsibility our position places us, with awe and respect. Before you leave your house in the morning to the clinic, prepare yourself for the day. Dispose your mind to change a life. Dispose yourself to save a life. This is a holistic process. It begins with the kind of prayer you make, the kind of wish you make, and the kind of thoughts you permit to take charge of your mind. You have a responsibility to communicate better. And for you to do that, you must be vigilant and take charge of every other aspect of your life.

PART THREE

HEAL

Healing is a natural restoration process built into the system of every life form. For healing to occur, there must be balance within the system of the lifeform. Balance is a state ensured by hemostasis. In humans, balance exists only when there is a synchronous alignment between the body, mind, and spirit. The process of creating balance begins in the mind. Hence healing here is referred to as a "communicated thought process". The work of a health provider is a vocation and not just a job. To carry out this vocation with utmost sincerity of purpose, the healthcare provider must adopt the virtues of a "healthcare giver," one who caters for the health of the patient holistically. "Holistic healthcare" is the means for achieving this.

CHAPTER EIGHT

HEALED BY FAITH

Under idyllic skies in southern California in April, a young athlete was filled with a wave of unbridled optimism, as he was about to race in a Palm Springs triathlon. Having successfully completed the swimming segment, his joy knew no bounds as he prepared for the biking portion of the race. However, something unexpected happened. If only the eyes can see beyond the visible, so many events will be avoided- no matter what it promises.

Now known as Dr Joe Dispenser, was merely 23 years old when this unfortunate incident happened. Having practiced so fearlessly hard for the triathlon, he was tragically run over by an SUV during the biking phase of the race.

Following a series of x-rays, tests, and scans, he discovered he had compression fractures in his spine, and injuries in the thoracic 8, 9, 10, 11, and 12 as well as the lumbar 1. The magnitude of the pain he experienced was beyond belief.

He was soon presented with an option - a major surgery to implant a Harrington rod. Somewhat a good option, at least he was sure to walk again. But aside from walking again, there was a looming fear, future gloom, and unsatisfaction lurking within the supposed better option. What could he do? Take it and suffer chronic pain forever? or reject it and appeal to the unknown?

Joe at this time, still young and daring, decided not to take the surgery, against professional advice and recommendations.

But the question was; could there be a chance for him? Could he possibly survive this without external help? He sure was going to regret he never took the surgery.

 Despite all warnings, Joe was driven from the hospital back home under the host of his two friends. Where he would work without relent on self-healing. Part of his strategies was first: to begin every day by reconstructing his spine, vertebra by vertebra. It sounds easy, but would it be that simple? For him to accomplish this goal, he had to be present at the moment without feeling sorry for himself or bursting into regret.

Joe was dead sure of what he wanted, and he created that reality in his mind through visualization. Imagining himself as completely healed, he meditated twice a day for two hours.

On several occasions, he lost it, and thoughts of a paralyzed existence kept stalking him. In his words "I realized back then that when crisis or trauma occurs, we spend too much of our attention and energy thinking about what we don't want instead of what we do want. During those first several weeks,

I was guilty of this tendency on what seemed like a moment-to-moment basis. In the middle of my meditations on creating the life I wanted with a fully healed spine, I would all of a sudden become aware that I'd been unconsciously thinking about what the surgeons had told me a few weeks prior: that I would probably never walk again."

Joe believed that at the core of each of us, lies a superior intelligence capable of accomplishing whatever we wish. He didn't stop. Soon, his imagined grievance began to vanish into thin air. This time his vision of a healed vertebra was longer and more detailed than before. The adjustment began to smooth out, with more noticeable changes in his physical state, and by nine and a half weeks after the accident, his life had fully returned to normal. As impossible as it may sound, Joe had no surgery to walk again.

The Process of Healing

Healing is the process of restoration of health from an unbalanced, diseased, damaged, or unvitalized organism. Nursing traditionally has been concerned with matters of healing, whereas medicine has historically been concerned with curing.

Healing occurs when an organism suffers physical damage or disease and the cell(s), organ, and biological system as a whole are repaired, and normal functioning is again restored. The process of medicine involves regenerating the body's cell(s) to replace damaged or necrotic tissue with useful, living new cells to reduce the size of the defective area. It can be done either through regeneration, where new cells form tissue similar to that which was originally there, or through repair, where injured tissue is repaired by forming scar tissue. Organs usually heal by combining both mechanisms.

In surgery, healing is more commonly referred to as recovery, and postoperative recovery is traditionally seen as

regaining function and being ready for discharge. The postoperative recovery process has been described as an energy*consuming process that decreases physical symptoms, attains emotional well-being, regains functions, and resumes normal activities.

Psychiatry and psychology define healing as the process by which neuroses and psychoses are resolved to such an extent that the client can lead a normal or fulfilling life without being overwhelmed by psychopathological phenomena. Psychotherapy, pharmaceutical treatment, and alternative approaches, including spiritual healing, can be a part of this process. The main thing is to restore the mind to optimal functionality.

Healing is also referred to in the context of grieving. When you suffer from psychological trauma, it is assumed that there is a wound the trauma causes in your mind. The emotional dislodgement brings about psychological neurosis that goes from anxiety to depression and possibly worse circumstances.

To restore the mind, a healing process has to happen. This sometimes can mean helping you forget the experience or reframing the experience totally. Both of which involve erasing or rewiring the neural pathways the memories have created in the brain.

Losing a loved one can be unbearable. As you can imagine, grief is difficult and we often wonder if the suffering will ever end. As humans, we go through a wide array of emotional experiences, including anger, confusion, and sadness.

According to psychiatrist Elisabeth Kübler-Ross, we go through five distinct stages of grief after losing a loved one: denial, anger, bargaining, depression, and finally acceptance. These five stages of grief are equally applicable whenever we suffer huge pain from grief. This process is perhaps a healing process that we go through to come to the point of acceptance where the pain no longer hunts us.

From the explanation so far, you can understand that healing is simply the restoration of a healthy state of being.

This can be achieved in any life form, and through any means that involves the proper balancing of the energy system in the body so that they can perform optimally.

Healing begins as a process to balance an unbalanced system. In a self-organizing system operating within the laws of physics and chemistry, healing begins the process of health restoration communicated through the energy forces that exist within the system.

Healing as A Communicated Thought Process

There is a complex system of processes involved in any kind of healing process. A close observation of all these processes shows that healing is not a carefree process. It is actually a methodic and calculated process. It involves the communication of different parts of a system to enable it to reorganize itself and restore the system to normalcy. In the body healing is at best a communicated thought process. By that, I mean communication of energy signals. It begins in the mind, then the brain being the physical tool of the mind coordinates the process and distribution of energy across the whole system of the body. For healing to occur the mind must be sound. And what makes a mind sound? To a large extent, the message it has over time received from outside.

It all begins with perception or belief

Providing scientific evidence to support a holistic approach to wellbeing and healthcare, Bruce Lipton sheds light on the mechanism underlying healing at a cellular level. He emphasizes that 'love' is the most healing emotion and the 'placebo effect' accounts for a substantial percentage of *any* drug's action, underscoring the significance of beliefs in health and sickness. According to him, as adults, we still believe in and act our lives out based on information we absorbed as children (pathetic indeed!). And the good news is, we can do something about the 'tape' our subconscious mind is playing, and change them NOW.

To show this let's begin with the most common places where we find healing. In a bodily wound. How does healing occur in a wound?

It is common knowledge that wounds heal. But sometimes we take the process that creates it for granted. A small cut can be cleaned and bandaged and you are good to go. Nonetheless, under that bandage (or in the open air) the body orchestrates a complex series of events that heal both large and small wounds.

The human body is a complex and remarkable machine, and the body's dynamic wound healing process provides an excellent example of how our various systems work together to repair and replace necrotic tissue. But how exactly, does the human body heal?

When the skin is injured, our body automatically sets in motion a series of events, known as the "cascade of healing," to repair the wound. During the cascade of healing, there are four overlapping phases: Hemostasis, Inflammation, Proliferation, and Maturation.

Phase 1: Hemostasis Phase

Hemostasis is the first phase of healing, which begins when an injury occurs. Its objective is to stop bleeding. As part of this phase, the body activates its emergency repair system, the blood clotting system, and forms a dam to block drainage. Platelets are activated and aggregated when they come into contact with collagen. At its center, thrombin initiates the formation of a fibrin mesh, which strengthens the platelet clumps into a stable clot.

Phase 2: Defensive/Inflammatory Phase

Phase 1 focuses primarily on coagulation, while Phase 2, or the Defensive/Inflammatory Phase, focuses on destroying bacteria and removing debris, creating a healthy wound bed for further healing.

Neutrophils, a type of white blood cell, enter the wound during Phase 2 to destroy bacteria and remove debris. It is common for these cells to reach their peak population between 24 and 48 hours after injury, and they drastically decrease after three days. White blood cells leave, and specialized cells called macrophages arrive to continue clearing debris. Additionally, these cells secrete growth factors and proteins that attract immune system cells to the wound to facilitate tissue repair. Usually, this phase lasts between four to six days and is characterized by edema, erythema (reddening of the skin), heat, and pain.

Phase 3: Proliferative Phase

Having been cleaned out, the wound enters the Proliferative Phase, where the focus is on filling and covering the wound.

In the proliferative phase, three phases are seen: 1) the wound is filled; 2) the margins are contracted, and 3) the wound is covered (epithelialization).

In the first stage, shiny, deep red granulation tissue fills the wound bed with connective tissue, and new blood vessels are formed. The wound margins contract and pull toward the center during contraction. From the wound bed or margins, epithelial cells emerge and migrate across the wound bed in a leapfrog pattern until the wound is covered with epithelium. The Proliferative phase is often between four and 24 days long.

Phase 4: Maturation Phase

In the Maturation phase, the new tissue gradually gains strength and flexibility. Collagen fibers reorganize, the tissue remodels and matures, and there is a general increase in tensile strength (though maximum strength is limited to 80% of pre-injury strength). Maturation lasts anywhere from 21 days to two years depending on the wound.

This remarkable and complex process of healing can be interrupted by local, emotional, and systemic factors, including moisture, infection, and maceration (local factors), age, nutritional status, also the state of mind and stress level which affects the functionality of the immune system to encourage repair (emotional factors) and finally the type of body that the patient possesses (systemic factors). If the right environment for healing is created, the human body has wondrous ways of healing and replacing devitalized tissue. The communication between cells of the body is so remarkable. If you understand the process, you will begin to appreciate why healing is a process of communication of energy signals.

A Vanderbilt University team of physicists and biologists used an ultrafast, ultraprecise laser to understand the nature of wound healing. Professor of Physics and Biological Sciences Shane Hutson and Associate Professor of Cell and Developmental Biology Andrea Page-McCaw targeted cells on the backs of fruit fly pupae that expressed a protein that fluoresced when calcium ions were present. Their findings are described in a paper titled "Multiple mechanisms drive calcium signal dynamics around laser induced epithelial wounds" published by the Biophysical Journal on Oct. 3. 2017.

By focusing a laser at a very small spot, the team of researchers created microscopic marks in the pupae's epithelial layer that could punch microscopic holes in individual cells (less than a millionth of a meter). "As a result, the damage the laser pulses produce is quite similar to a puncture wound surrounded by a crush wound—blunt force trauma in forensic terms—so our observations should apply to most common wounds," said first author Erica Shannon, a doctoral student in developmental biology. As Shannon explains further: "It turns out cells have a number of different ways to signal injury. This may allow them to differentiate between different kinds of wounds."

A complex series of calcium signals are generated in the tissue surrounding a wound, as shown by the experiments:

First, there is a rapid influx of calcium into the cells immediately around the wound. The footprint of the cavitation bubble matches this. Within cells, calcium concentrations are much lower than those in extracellular fluid. Researchers suggest that this influx occurs due to micro-tears in cell membranes ripped open by the force of the micro-explosion because of the rapidity with which it occurs (less than a tenth of a second);

A short-lived, short-ranged wave then spreads through neighboring healthy cells. The bigger the wound, the more quickly it spreads. The wave's speed suggests that it travels through gap junctions and is either composed of calcium ions or some other type of small signaling molecule.

A second wave appears about 45 seconds after wounding. The second wave spreads considerably farther but moves much more slowly than the first. This implies that it is spread by larger molecules, most likely signaling proteins, which diffuse more slowly than ions. The second wave only occurs when cells are killed, not when they are just damaged, suggesting that it is dependent on the extent of the damage.

The first two waves spread across the tissue relatively symmetrically. However, after the second wave, the high calcium concentration area begins to release flares-directional streams of calcium influx that spread far into the surrounding tissue. Each flare lasts for ten seconds, and new flares continue to occur for more than 30 minutes after an injury.

This process of energy diffusion and spread within the body once the damage is incurred begins the healing process. The spread of waves is the spread of energy frequency across the body. It is the process of energy communication across different parts of the body beginning with the implicated cells to tissues and organs.

In principle, this mechanism of the healing process is the same across all health breakdowns. Once the system breaks down the process of restoration begins immediately. There's a naturally self-organizing system that automates the healing process so that it is auto intelligent. However, this automated self-organizing system can be disrupted when there's a disorder within the system. Like a disease or diabetes. People with uncontrolled diabetes develop poor circulation as a result. As circulation slows down, blood moves more slowly, which makes it more difficult for the body to deliver nutrients to wounds. As a result, the injuries heal slowly, or may not heal at all. This disruption can cause the system not to heal automatically.

But this disruption is not only caused by physical disruptors like diabetics. Psychological factors can equally contribute to the disruption of the system. This is seen when there's an emotional breakdown coming from anxiety or a highly nervous situation which could lead to many "disbalances" within the human body, ranging from mild fear to depression. A functional and properly working immune system will slow the process of healing to go on normally. But when your immune system is disrupted either through local physical factors like shortage of vital hormones or by trauma caused by emotional "disbalance". It could result in the delay or total obstruction of the healing process depending on the degree of the tissue damage that has been secured.

In the light of this understanding, it is not out of place to say that fear can disrupt within the system, anxiety can affect the system, panic can equally cause that. And if we trace the source of these nonphysical disruptors we can find that poor communication would be hugely implicated. How?

The Role of Communication in Healing

Health begins with communication as healing begins with communication. The process of healing as you have seen is an internal system communication between cells, tissues, and organs. As it is internally, so it is externally. The process of communication begins externally as it is induced by external factors.

This is where clinician-patient communication comes in. As a healthcare giver, it is the responsibility of the clinician to

communicate health to the patient. The manner of communication of the clinician imparts directly or indirectly in all aspects of the healing process. It affects the healing process in ways the actors have never thought about. Let me explore some of it to let you have a glimpse of the full picture.

The literature of medicine and healthcare is replete with studies and evidence of the direct and indirect relationship between communication and healing.

Medical Research indicates that features of clinician-patient communication can predict health outcomes weeks and months after the consultation. For example, talk itself, can be therapeutic. It can help in lessening the patient's anxiety and providing comfort.

More often clinician-patient communication influences health outcomes via a more indirect route. This happens on two levels: proximal outcomes and intermediate outcomes.

Proximal outcomes of the interaction include patient understanding, trust, and clinician-patient agreement. These affect intermediate outcomes (e.g., increased adherence, better self-care skills) which, in turn, affect health and well-being.

In their work... Richard L Street and his colleagues Gregory Makoul, Neeraj K Arora, and Ronald M Epstein explain there are seven pathways through which communication can lead to better health. These include:

1. Increased access to care,

2. Greater patient knowledge and shared understanding,

3. Higher quality medical decisions,

4. Enhanced therapeutic alliances,

5. Increased social support,

6. Patient agency and empowerment, and

7. Better management of emotions.

Cross-sectional studies have shown that communication behaviors between physicians and patients affect health outcomes. As one example, the characteristics of patient-centered communication-including clear explanations, compassion, and involvement in decision-making - have been linked to decreases in blood pressure, anxiety, and organ damage among patients with systemic lupus erythematosus, and a better quality of life among breast cancer patients.

In a paper by Richard L Street, his colleagues Gregory Makoul, Neeraj K Arora, and Ronald M Epstein they admonished that researchers "must also recognize and try to account for the fact that outcomes, especially those related to cancer and chronic disease, are likely less influenced by a single clinician-patient encounter, and more by the cumulative effect of the patient's communication over time with their physicians, others on the care team, families, and friends. These points to the overlapping effects of communication in other settings and in the long term."

CHAPTER NINE

THE RELATIONSHIPS BETWEEN COMMUNICATION AND IMPROVED HEALTH

What Improves Physical Health?

Physical health status includes pain and other symptoms, disease markers (e.g., hemoglobin A1C, blood pressure, weight, prostate-specific antigen), functional capacity (e.g., ability to walk), and subjective self-ratings of health. Richard L. Street et al identify that "there are essentially four types of therapeutic regimens that lead to improved physical health — chemical (e.g., medication), mechanical (e.g., surgery), behavioral (e.g.,

smoking cessation, diet), and psychological (e.g., placebo effects, cognitive therapy). For example, a patient could experience improved physical health because he or she received medication that controlled the disease, received necessary surgical intervention (e.g., a stent), adopted healthier exercise routines, or believed - based on what he was told - that the treatment was effective. Thus, following the last instance, communication could lead to better physical health. Conversations between clinician and patient can help to identify the correct diagnosis and appropriate treatment plan, which can lead to following through with treatment or self-care, and/or affected patients' health beliefs."

Let's Look at What Improves the Psychosocial Aspects of Health?

As Richard and his colleagues explain "Psychosocial health is a function of the degree to which an individual has more positive beliefs and feelings, harbors fewer negative beliefs and

feelings (e.g., worry, anger, anxiety, fear, despair), and has a well-functioning social network. Psychological wellbeing, vitality, self-efficacy, and social functioning are typically measured by patient (sometimes family) self-report. Positive psychosocial outcomes can be the direct result of communicative encounters (including those with clinicians) from which patients feel known, validated, hopeful, worthy, reassured, and comforted and indirectly through diagnosis and treatment of mental disorders (e.g., depression) and reinforcing social support".

Communication Pathways to Improved Health Outcomes

Richard L. Street explains in their paper that identifying the mode of communication that influences health and wellbeing is important to understand how communication may improve or deteriorate health outcomes. The pathways through which communication can impact healing and health are twofold -

direct and indirect. It is direct for example, in the instance of verbal communication.

Talk is therapeutic. When a physician validates a patient's perspective or expresses empathy, it can enhance psychological well-being - fewer negative emotions (e.g., fear, anxiety) and more positive ones (e.g., hope, optimism, and self-worth). Talk can also affect physical symptoms. A study found empathic communication lowered physiological arousal and pain among patients with symptoms of irritable bowel syndrome. Finally, nonverbal communication such as touch and voice tone may also improve wellbeing directly by reducing anxiety.

Richard and his colleagues explain that the role of communication in ensuring health is indispensable. Analyzing further how this can be achieved through direct and indirect means, the authors stated it in such a way that I can't help but cite them in full:

> However, in most cases, communication
> affects health through a more indirect or
> mediated   route   through   proximal

outcomes of the interaction (e.g., satisfaction with care, motivation to adhere, trust in the clinician and system, self-efficacy in self-care, clinician-patient agreement, and shared understanding) that could then affect health or that could contribute to the intermediate outcomes (e.g., adherence, self-management skills, social support) that lead to better health. For example, a clinician's clear explanations and expressions of support could lead to greater patient trust and understanding of treatment options (proximal outcomes). This in turn may facilitate patient follow-through with recommended therapy (an intermediate outcome), which in turn improves a particular health outcome (e.g., disease control, emotional well-being). Or, patient participation in the consultation could help the physician better understand the patient's needs and preferences as well as discover possible misconceptions the patient might have about treatment options. The physician can then communicate risk information in a way the patient understands which in turn could lead to a mutually agreed upon, higher-quality decision that best matches the patient's circumstances. In a recent National Cancer Institute monograph, we proposed that clinician-patient communication can contribute to improved health through at least seven 'pathways'—access to needed care, increased patient knowledge and shared understanding, enhancing therapeutic alliances (among clinicians, patient, and family), enhancing emotional self-management, activating social support and advocacy resources, increasing the quality of medical decisions(e.g., informed, clinically sound, concordant with patient values, and mutually endorsed), and enabling patient agency (self-efficacy and empowerment). Although these pathways were explored with respect to cancer care, they are certainly applicable to other health conditions as well.

There's no doubt that communication plays a big role in improving health. Mastering the art of communication is therefore not an optional skill. The art of communication is an art of influence. You influence the patient's decision, mindset, actions, and health outcomes. It starts from the mind then to the body. In performing your art of communication remember that the patient is coming from somewhere. A place from where she has received and downloaded the information and thoughts that have made her sick. A toxic environment that has caused an internal imbalance that has resulted in sickness. Your job is to restore her to a state of balance by communicating peace and health. To understand how to do this, follow me through the final part of this book where I will show you the relationship between balance and healing. And how communication is the link between both.

CHAPTER TEN

ENERGY BALANCE AND HEALING

Every system in life from the unicellular amoeba to our planet earth requires an inbuilt mechanism for ensuring balance. Earth-atmosphere energy balance is achieved when solar energy balances the energy, that the Earth loses back into space. Thus, the Earth maintains a stable average temperature and therefore a stable climate. The contractile vacuoles of amoebas help them maintain internal balance through what is called osmoregulation. It does this by shunting excess water and waste products to the contractile vacuole for storage. When the vacuole is full, it violently contracts and expels the water and waste.

As James O Hill, and his colleagues explain in a paper on *"The Importance of Energy Balance"*, "The concept of energy balance is based on the fundamental thermodynamic principle that energy cannot be destroyed, and can only be gained, lost, or stored by an organism. Energy balance is defined as the state achieved when the energy intake equals energy expenditure. This concept may be used to demonstrate how body weight will change over time in response to changes in energy intake and expenditure. When the body is in energy balance, bodyweight is stable. Humans take in energy through the intake of food and drink, and expend energy through the resting metabolic rate (RMR)—the thermic effect (TEF) of food and physical activity. The RMR is the energy expenditure required for maintaining normal body functions and homeostasis."

In a healthy human body, the body performs all the work necessary to maintain itself by using what is termed "living processes," which include the excretion of waste and inhalation of oxygen to release energy from sugar. In addition, the body uses homeostasis to maintain balance - it makes just the right number of new cells to replace worn-out ones, and just the right amount of hormones to signal a reaction when needed.

Health is homeostasis. It is an internal feedback system that keeps our body's chemistry balanced so our organs function smoothly and efficiently together. It is the disruption of homeostasis that leads to illness, which is treated by medicine. However, some medicine sometimes disrupts one homeostatic mechanism while adjusting another, leading to more sickness and more medicine. This is why medicines are so profitable but have so many side effects and adverse reactions. It is therefore advisable for healthcare practitioners to minimize medicine and maximize holistic factors, such as lifestyle, diet, exercise, education, recreation, and relationships - all of which find themselves in the basket of effective communication.

Homeostasis is a state of balance between biochemical and physiological pathways that are maintained through constant adjustment. A good example of homeostasis is the maintenance of constant blood pressure in the human body through adjustment of the hormonal, neuromuscular, and cardiovascular systems within their normal range. This allows a person's blood pressure to remain stable despite changes in the environment and changes in their activities and positions. Similarly, other homeostatic mechanisms keep the body temperature within a narrow range.

Your body has an internal mechanism that ensures that there is a homeostatic balance from the cellular level to the level of tissues, organs, and the whole body. A homeostatic balance on a general body level is what we call good health.

Homeostasis as a mechanism for the maintenance of steady states in the body by coordinated physiological mechanisms works through the communication of the body's internal interdependent processes. Cellular communication is essential to integrate and coordinate the systems of the body so they can participate in different functions. At the heart of homeostatic function and coordination is communication.

Communication here is what is known as cell signaling. How does it work and what's the process involved?

Cell Signaling:

Cellular communication is essential for integrating and coordinating body systems so they can perform their functions. Cell-cell signaling involves the transmission of a signal from a sending cell to a receiving cell. An example is the conduction of an electric signal from one nerve cell to another or a muscle cell. In this case, the signaling molecule is a neurotransmitter.

What does cell signaling have to do with the homeostasis of cells? Homeostasis involves cell signaling because homeostasis makes the cell able to behave and correctly respond to the receptor. Hormones are transported through the circulatory

system and then delivered to nearby tissues. Hormones can be sent to cells' receptors to signal another change in the body. Different body functions are regulated by these hormones.

How else besides cell signaling, do cells maintain homeostasis? Through Vacuoles and chloroplasts. Organisms respond to changes in their environment through behavior and physiological mechanisms. In behavior mechanisms, we can find avoidance and compensation. Avoidance is the ability to avoid things that cause distress physically or mentally; Compensation is finding ways to compensate for a weakness in one area by gaining strength in another. An example of a physiological mechanism would be a temperature change. When a bird gets cold, its brain sends a message that winter may be approaching. The bird will then fly south so it will stay warm and not freeze. They are responding to a signal they are receiving.

Communication is at the heart of behavior and psychological mechanisms. Communication works together with the environment.

Providing Stability for Cells

A cell is the unit of life; it is the building block of life. Our cells, like all living organisms, need to be maintained to keep us alive. Living organisms exist in two environments:

The external environment, the planet on which we find ourselves, Earth;

The internal environment, the one beneath our skin.

The external environment is constantly changing. Variables (such as temperature, water levels, air pressure, oxygen levels, and nitrogen levels) can be measured, but they cannot be changed. Our internal environment is impacted by these changes, but for life to continue, our internal environment must remain stable.

Our internal environment can be impacted by physiological mechanisms. Cells in the body are composed of chemicals, such as proteins, which can only survive under very specific conditions. Eggs, for example, consist mainly of a protein called albumin, which becomes solid when heated. Albumin is also found in our bodies, and our bodies are equally susceptible to temperature changes. Enzymes, which allow bodily reactions to happen, are made of proteins. In the case of any changes to the internal conditions, the enzymes would not function, and neither would we: our entire metabolism, the chemistry of our cells, all would cease to function.

Proteins and cells are both highly sensitive to changes in variables in their internal (and external) environments. Cells must be maintained at certain temperatures, pH (a measure of hydrogen ion concentration revealing our acid-base balance), osmotic balance (the balance between water and solutes), and energy levels (sugar and oxygen). The cells of a human are part of a vast community - a typical adult human consists of trillions of them - and therefore they need to communicate to know what's happening. All of this is part of our internal environment.

Our internal environment can be equally impacted by behavior mechanisms communicated through the external environment. The external environment communicates to the internal environment. The relationship of communication is what happens with phenotype and genotype. Phenotypes are observable traits of an individual, such as height, eye color, and blood type. The genotype is the genetic contribution to the phenotype. Certain traits are largely determined by a person's genotype, while others are largely determined by their environment. While genotype is the internal, phenotype is the evidence of the influence of the external environment.

The receptors in the body receive information about a change of state in variables that it monitors, and send signals to the brain for coordination, so all the information can be integrated into one place. Next, a response message is sent out to encourage a specific response or behavior. The response can be electrical (sent via the nervous system) or chemical (sent via the endocrine system) and it prompts a change, or effect, to return our internal conditions to an optimal state. This is brought about by organs or cells known as 'effectors' because they "effect" a response.

Changing environments

The external and internal environments are constantly changing. It may get hotter or colder outside. Accidents could cause trauma. Noise could cause anxiety or phonophobia. Traumatic events could equally cause anxiety. We lose water in the body through evaporation; food changes the pH of the body, and cells die and require replacement in the appropriate quantity. To offset the effects of these changes, the internal environment is monitored and compensated for.

Despite its inability to control the external environment, the body can regulate its internal environment to react appropriately to changes in all variables. The kidneys regulate salt, water, and pH; blood carries heat to all parts of the body, oxygen to the cells, and removes carbon dioxide from them. Homoeostasis is responsible for all of these regulations.

The Foundation of Health

Claude Bernard first proposed the concept of homeostasis in 1865, and Walter Cannon named it in 1926. Often, it is described as "the maintenance of a stable internal environment". However, student health professionals seldom find this definition useful as it is with many theories they learn in medical school. The real challenge comes when they qualify as practitioners. The lack of a clear understanding of the connection between homeostasis and health becomes a problem. The first step in understanding the patient journey and clinical decision-making begins with the understanding that homeostasis is the cornerstone of health, and its restoration, the foundation of clinical care.

In homeostasis, physiological processes (what the body does) are linked to its cells (what the body is made of). The body's homeostatic mechanisms ensure that variables remain within normal ranges, allowing cells to survive and thrive. Physiologically, homeostasis ensures that the internal environment is stabilized and normal. Homoeostasis uses chemical and biological processes for self-maintenance.

Adjusting Change

Humans are dynamic beings. Throughout the day, the body fluctuates based on internal and external triggers: it gets hotter and colder, sweatier and dehydrated, energetic and tired. Aside from physical triggers, psychological and emotional factors also affect the functioning of the system. Like when a loved one is harmed, financial issues, relationship fights. These highly charged emotional triggers can disrupt the system. As long as we are healthy, we rarely notice these changes because we can adjust our variables to put ourselves back in a safe place:

drinking hot drinks or cold drinks; eating or stopping food; active or resting. Changes in behavior are motivated by internal processes that seek to prevent us from getting too hot, too cold, too dehydrated, or too full of energy, thus restoring us to a safe state.

As the external and internal environments are changing all the time, the body needs to keep the variables of its internal environment within ranges that are tolerable for its cells, and this is done by homeostasis. Homoeostasis, which allows the body to maintain its internal environment independently of clinical support, is a measure of health. Ill health is when the body is no longer homoeostatic and clinical intervention is an attempt to restore homeostasis.

This is where communication comes in.

Effective communication begins in the mind. A Patient who is not healthy in the mind cannot manifest a healthy state of being. Homeostatic pattern regulation will be impeded. Your job primarily as a healthcare giver is to help the patient get to this primary state of being. It is from this primary state that the patient can then move to improve other functions in their body.

Cell communication happens through the process of cell signaling. It allows the homeostasis to perform optimally in the state of normalcy when all the requirements needed to set them in motion are in place. To a large extent, poor communication within the cells can hamper this.

Cell signaling works with hormones and neurotransmitters; these processes could be hampered if the emotional and mental state of the patient is jeopardized through stress. Under stress, the autonomic nervous and endocrine systems respond by producing the hormones epinephrine, norepinephrine, and cortisol. The result of this hormone production is a cascade of physiological reactions that make up the stress response. These changes make up the fight-or-flight response, production of β-endorphin (the body's natural pain killer), and increased acuity of the senses which prepares the body to cope with the stressor. The excessive release of these hormones can hamper the healing process and disrupt the homeostatic balance in the body that ensures health. The job of the clinician who is a healthcare giver is to get the patient in the state of balance, first before beginning every other treatment. This process should begin with proper communication. Healing is first communicated before health is achieved. As a clinician, your main concern shouldn't be on the body of the patient only, but even more importantly on the psychology of your patient. Your job is to communicate healing in your words and actions. You're not just a clinician, you are a healthcare giver.

An understanding of homeostasis and the states that are optimal for body cells can be useful in healthcare. This can be done empirically through the observation of humans in health and ill health, and scientifically using objective measurement. It can help healthcare providers to understand the usefulness of effective communication. How so?

When a continuous perturbation persists, the homeostatic response does not completely restore the regulated variable to its original value. This is known as an error signal. It is used to maintain the homeostatic response. Homeostatic mechanisms with higher precision, result in a smaller error signal and lower fluctuations in the setting of the variable.

Homeostatic balance is regulated using three types of feedback systems. The first is a negative feedback system. This is the situation where an increase or decrease in a variable being regulated leads to responses moving the variable in the opposite direction. The second is a positive feedback system. This occurs when a disruption leads to a series of events that lead to an even greater disturbance. By driving a system away from its set point, it moves it away from its normal state. Such resetting may be adaptive and serve as the body's defense mechanism. Setpoints may also change rhythmically.

Feedforward regulation anticipates changes in variable values, improves homeostatic response speed, and minimizes deviation from setpoint values. The regulation may involve external detectors or a learning process

Communication Is a Homeostatic Enabler in The Body

As a healthcare giver, you need to understand this communication system within the body and model your medical communication approach after it.

In interfacing with your patients, assess the situation at hand and understand when to use negative feedback in your communication with the patient to drive healing in your patient. This feedback begins with verbal communication but equally extends to both nonverbal communication and other steps you take in restoring their health.

You must learn to understand what constitutes negative feedback and other kinds of feedback. Negative feedback could be found in even seemingly affirmative statements like "Yeah, you can do whatever you like"! You should do what's

best for you! Negative feedback can also be based on the context and the type of response given in such peculiar situations.

Accessing a situation and critically judging it before acting is key to communicating health to the patient.

When a patient is off the course of catastrophe sometimes they need negative feedback to bring them back on course. Important way doctors use in accessing the level of health of a patient is by checking their vital signs. Monitoring vital signs is an objective way to assess homeostasis and to know whether patients' health is improving or deteriorating Through these objective measurements, clinicians can implement potentially lifesaving interventions that will regain homeostasis. It is important to note that achieving health in a patient doesn't require only the medical application of drugs and procedures but a psychological analysis and communication of the language of healing can equally be effective. Sometimes parents give negative feedback to make their children behave. It is called "Vitamin N". Saying no to the child. Saying no when they request something they lust over just to help them build the character of delayed gratification. Another method could be the use of negotiated minimal force. These methods can be adapted in healthcare to help the patient get back on track. But you must assess the situation to know when best to use this feedback mechanism.

There's also a need to understand when to use positive feedback to counterbalance the health of your patient when their system has been imbalanced by negative feedback. Using words of encouragement could help a patient heal faster when they are in pain. Showing acts of kindness like checking up on them even when they don't expect it. Gifting them best "wishes cards", offering meaningful support in any meaningful way, can help the patient in their healing process.

Finally, you must be proactive in relating to your patient's health by using a feedforward approach to anticipate and communicate to your patient possible hazardous lifestyles and activities that they should avoid or stop engaging in.

Health is a holistic approach and to ensure a healthy state you must be circumspective in your approach. Knowing when to use these three steps in attending to the needs of your patient will help a lot in helping your patient heal and stay healthy.

CHAPTER ELEVEN

COMMUNICATING BALANCE AND HEALTH

The state of things flows from outside to inside. Health is communicated from outside to inside. From the external environment to the internal environment. The external environment communicates signals to the internal environment and the body's internal mechanism tries to adjust its operations accordingly to maintain balance. As a healthcare giver, when a patient visits you, it is your responsibility to take charge of their external environment so that you can influence their internal environment by

communicating health. But how can you do this? To do this you must understand the concept and role of a healthcare giver.

Throughout this book, I have been using the concept of the "healthcare giver". But what does it mean in the context of thinking, communicating, and healing? Let's find out.

Who Is a Healthcare Giver?

In its simplest terms, a healthcare giver is someone who restores health by communicating healing.

What does this mean? The job of every healthcare provider is to ensure that patients get holistic healthcare not just to have the specific issue that they are afflicted with. This is because no health issue is a consequence of one problem. All health issues are holistic problems that encompass a myriad of other issues, including body, mental and spiritual. You will appreciate the truth-value of this statement when you understand what the meaning of the word health means.

The statutory definition of the word health means "the condition of being sound in body, mind, and spirit. It means a condition in which someone or something is thriving or doing health". From this, you can understand that the word health connotes wellbeing. There cannot be a state of wellbeing without a balance of factors and elements in health components - Understand that health components are body, mind, and spirit - For this to happen there must be a steady state in the internal environment of your body. There must be equilibrium. Steady-state and equilibrium are distinct conditions. A steady-state is a condition that does not change over time. This is the condition that is maintained with homeostasis, while equilibrium represents a balance between opposing forces. This creates balance across the internal environment and the external environment, both of which have opposing forces. For a steady state and equilibrium to be achieved there must be a coordinated relationship between the body, mind, and spirit. When this coordinated relationship is achieved, a balance that results in health is achieved.

A healthcare giver is anyone who restores health by ensuring the balance of the body, mind, and spirit.

However, for any clinician to achieve this, they will have to combine life virtues with medical competence.

Genuine Love for Your Patient:

The rule for a clinician is that he or she must have a genuine concern and love for the patient. And this love must be manifested in the virtues of care, compassion, and kindness. A clinician cannot display these qualities if he or she doesn't love what they do. Love for what you do comes from a sense of purpose. It is this sense of purpose that creates a vocation out of your medical job. Like I have explained in the first part of this book, as a clinician you must ensure that what you are and how you are, align. Only when your personality aligns with your medical knowledge will you be able to deliver the work of a healthcare giver. This alignment can only come from a sense of vocation.

If you make your medical job your vocation you will approach it with a sense of purpose. Then your concern for every patient who steps into your presence would be how to make them whole and restored.

A genuine love for your patient creates a sense of urgency with which you would attend to the issues of your patient. It creates a sense of attentiveness that allows you to pay close attention and be hyper-alert.

By paying attention to the needs of your patient you will go beyond what is prescribed by the books, to what is needed to help your patient heal. These books prescribe the minimum standard of operation not the ideal mode of operation. When you approach your work with this kind of mindset you will soon begin to notice that you can now pay attention to the three key important aspects of your patient's health.

The healthcare giver uses the method of holistic healthcare to communicate health

Holistic therapy is a healthcare approach that focuses on caring for the individual as a system not as singular parts.

In my research of this topic I came across many topics

The approach of holistic healthcare founded within the principles and approach of holistic therapy begins with the understanding that health is a result of the sound balance between the body, mind, and spirit. This comes from the understanding that as humans our nature is triune.

The Body:

This refers to the physical body with all its physiological processes. The relationship between the internal environment and the external environment. Here the healthcare giver attends to the body itself using medicine and other physiotherapy enhancing methods. The healthcare giver also looks at the external environment and how it's impacting the internal environment.

However as critical as this part of health is to our wellbeing, it is not the only thing that careers well-being. Well-being can only be created in balance. And that is why the body has to coordinate with the mind.

The Mind:

The second part of holistic healthcare deals with the mind. This involves psychotherapy. This focuses on communicating healing thoughts and ideas to the mind so that the mind of the patient can nurture and cultivate these thoughts. By nurturing these thoughts in the internal monologue the patient can reframe the internal language which would to a large extent influence the internal environment of a patient. This is possible because internal language sets the nature of energy for the internal environment.

There's no doubt about the fact that the state of your mind affects the state of your body. For when you are angry your body releases toxic hormones like adrenaline and cortisol. These hormones make you stressed, which in turn impacts your cells, tissues, and organs. Your wellbeing is disorganized and your internal environment loses its set point. In this situation, your body works to try to restore your balance through the process of homeostasis. If healthy thoughts and ideas are communicated to your mind using either verbal or non-verbal means, your brain instructs the pineal gland to secrete serotonin which makes you happy, and dopamine which jolts you to act. Depending on the situation and quality of thought in progress.

Your job as a healthcare giver is to understand the state of mind of your patient before you administer any medicine. You must try to understand their personality type, understand their psychosocial influence (environmental conditioning). This enables you to understand the impact of their external environment.

Using this psychoanalysis to understand the state of their mind allows you to be better informed before checking their vital signs to understand their internal environment. By combining knowledge of these two, you come a step closer to the use of holistic medicine for restoring the health of your patient.

Spirit:

The mention of spirituality should not be mistaken for religiosity. Spirituality is simply the connection to the state of higher consciousness by a sense of meaning. Every human needs a sense of meaning to thrive. Meaning is a sense of purpose and vision. A sense of why gives us hope and the reason to move on. A sense of something higher than others, whether real or imagined, but often imagined. Some people find this sense of meaning in their nation, some find it in their group, some find it in a social cause they fight for, others find it in their religion, others find it in sports and yet others find it in music or social group. No human can survive without a sense of meaning and purpose, Science has shown that we are actually wired to seek it. The nucleus accumbens is the part of our brain is dedicated to this. The nucleus accumbens core is involved in the cognitive processing of motor function related to reward and reinforcement and the regulation of slow-wave sleep. But specifically, the core encodes new motor programs which facilitate the acquisition of a given reward in the future. With its built-in reward mechanism, it energies us to act with a sense of purpose.

If you stimulate some parts of the brain with a transcranial magnetic stimulator it will create mystical and religious experiences based on which one is wired through conditioning and association to find meaning. Although there is no single "God spot" in the brain, feelings of self-transcendence are associated with reduced electrical activity in the right parietal lobe, a structure located above the right ear

Helping a patient align their body and mind with their spirit helps them heal faster. In communicating with your patients, you should help them reconnect back to their sense of meaning. Irrespective of where they get it from. By reconnecting patients to their sense of spirituality, you create hope in them. And so they have a reason for living. By seeing a reason for leaving, their mind and body work in tandem with their spiritual meaning to create balance in their internal environment for health to be restored.

Connecting patients to their sense of meaning or spirituality equally help them to find meaning in their external environment, thereby helping them to exercise a level of control over their environment. A factor very difficult to control yet has a huge consequence on our internal health.

For example, if you belong to a school of thought that believes that God has given you the earth to make whatever you wish. That everything happens for a reason that works in your favor. This kind of sense of meaning in time shifts your mindset in the way you interpret events that happen every day. You tend to have a more positive mindset that tries to rationalize even oppressive situations, to see the good in them even when there's none. While this might have its consequences, it tends to make your internal environment less hypertensive.

A sense of meaning and purpose helps you create a harmonic balance between your body and mind which brings health.

Your work as a healthcare giver is to create the conditions necessary to make your interactions with your patient go through these three processes. Only when you engage this holistic healthcare approach will you start seeing a meaningful improvement in the overall wellbeing of your patient. If you truly love and care for your patient, you will do these.

CONCLUSION

As Forrest Gump said, "Life is like a box of chocolates: you never know what you are going to get." In life, unforeseen circumstances can suddenly change one's role from a giver to a receiver; from a clinician to a patient. When a medical care provider suddenly becomes a patient and seeks medical care in the health care field, a lot of psychological changes take place that can alter the existing perspectives of that medical care provider with regards to the general health care delivery system.

I know from firsthand experience what it feels like to wear a hat: both for a clinician and a patient. After many years of practicing as a family nurse practitioner and enjoying good

health for most of my adult years, I suddenly discovered that I needed to have surgery for the repair of an abdominal hernia and the removal of an exceptionally large fibroid that had made it quite challenging for me to bend down without excruciating pain. In 2013, I underwent a major abdominal surgery and was unable to return to work for five months following the surgery. During this period of recovery, I traded my clinician hat for that of a patient. Although I believed I had always efficiently interacted with several of my patients through my professional years, I sincerely felt for the first time what it really meant to be a patient. As an active mother of four girls, I was terrified of the unknown that is typically associated with surgical routines requiring general anesthesia. So many questions flooded my mind. "Will I still be okay when I wake up? Who will care for my family as I recover?" (Thanks to my loving husband that issue was taken care of, but it still did not make me worry any less!)

Following the surgery, I realized that I was equally terrified of the recovery process, which involved follow-up tests, scans,

doctor's appointments, and more. It was during this recovery process that it finally clicked for me. I concluded that as a patient, there is a train of thought process and expected behaviors that will promote the development of a productive and trusting relationship with clinicians. As a clinician, I have always known that I must abide by certain codes and ethics in order to provide optimal care to my patients. But it was not until I spent a great deal of time as a patient in the health care system that it dawned on me that a trusting relationship cannot be successfully achieved in a unilateral format by either the patient or the clinician. It is a joint venture and a two-way street. Both parties must be willing to hold each other to a higher standard of conduct and participate wholeheartedly in the process of developing a successful clinician-patient relationship. I am happy to say that with the help of my wonderful doctors, and surely by the grace of God, I made a successful recovery and am back to caring for my patients, but not before I learned some valuable lessons that now help me better relate to my patients.

My experience in the hospital as a patient helped me appreciate even more my work as a healthcare provider. I understood that the work of a healthcare provider is not just a job but a vocation and mandate to restore health. This realization enabled me to approach my work differently. It allowed me to understand that my place in the healthcare setting is special and I had to treat it so. It turned on in me the light of compassion and kindness towards patients that I meet every day at work.

You see, when a patient comes into your office to meet you, they come to you openly and vulnerable. Irrespective of what kind of attitude they might present as a result of their personality type and mindset, you must understand that they are in pain. They need solace and succor. Even when they are angry, they need help; sad they need consolation; insulting they need attention; hostile they need understanding, talkative they need a listener, impatient they need a patient-clinician. They need a healthcare giver. One who can understand their pulse and their state even when they are unable to communicate them.

We often fail to understand that true communication comes from the heart, it is evidenced when you can see beyond the veil of what your interlocutor is saying to how they feel. Sometimes expecting our patient, or interlocutor to say exactly as they feel might not be possible for them. Sometimes they lack the language to articulate their feeling and emotions. It is left for you as one who understands communication to listen beyond what is being said and see beyond what is presented to understand the real needs of your patient or interlocutor.

The ability to do this comes not just from learning how to communicate effectively but by learning to show courage in the face of fear. At the heart of effective communication are courage and focus. Without courage, you cannot muster the will to say what needs to be said, when it needs to be said. Without courage, we cannot develop the compassion to hear the needs of others. Sometimes we are too afraid to listen to the needs of others. We feel we don't have the capacity, time, or resources to help. Sometimes we feel the other person may take advantage of us. We hear stories of people who have been

hurt by strangers they opened their arms to. Sometimes we are scared of reaching out because we feel unworthy. Or we feel others might not tolerate our differences and uniqueness.

All of these feelings, and emotions create bias, prejudice, and hatred. All of which are caused by fear. But fear isn't necessarily as bad as you may think it to be. Fear in itself can be a useful or destructive emotion depending on how you decide to use it. To understand the role of fear in our lives I ventured into the works of the renowned philosopher and the award-winning Fearist Osinakachi Akuma Kalu. In his book "Success Mantra" he explained the role of courage in overcoming fear so well that it requires a full citation:

> To combat fear, one demands intellectual courage. Begin to think of risks as opportunities not dangers, as stepping stones not stumbling blocks. To combat fear properly, you have to fight it out from your mind first. It is more of internal than external combat. Seek always to know the reality behind the phenomenon that you are afraid of. Seek enlightenment on the subject matter of your fear and fear will

immediately disappear once the light of true knowledge of things comes to your mind. It is our wrong beliefs and ignorance about the realities of life which give so much power and momentum to these fears to destroy us intellectually. Once the true knowledge dawns and consciousness awakens from its deep slumber in us, fear melts away on its own. Fear cannot stand up against an enlightened or awakened rational soul. Ken Oguejiofor was of this view when he wrote: 'Each time you seek out the features of fear you find out that it has a face behind the face. Eventually, you are led to the truth, and it is only the truth that can liberate you from the shackles of fear. Courage is the strength of the mind which enables people to be firm and resolute in the face of dangers or adverse circumstances without giving way to fear. Real courage does not mean never being afraid. It means doing what has to be done in spite of being afraid.'

We need the courage to summon the power to communicate and help others heal. My intention in this book has been to help you understand that communication within healthcare needs not to be a hassle. If you as a healthcare provider and patient can understand the relationship between what you think and what you express in any fashion, then you have received the enlightenment and power of restoration buried within you as a human. My hope and prayer for you are that you discover the hidden power of healing through your communication within and without.

I would like to hear from you after you have read this book. You can write at nonyetochiaghanya.com Feel free to share your testimonies of how this book has impacted your life and those around you. I encourage you also to gift a copy of this book to the people you care most about. Together we can create a healthy culture built on love, understanding, and effective communication. Life begins with communication and ends in its absence, burn the candle of life in your family, community, and workplace by keeping the knowledge and freedom that comes with effective communication. Leave a legacy by thinking clearly, communicating effectively, and healing holistically.

You can visit my website at www.nonyetochi.com to learn about my 30-year journey to effective communication. There you'll also find my other books, guidebooks, and courses where I share tips for effective communication.

I have an upcoming program called self-authoring suite for effective communication, this year 2021. This program offers you the chance to practice all the principles I have laid out in this book. You have the opportunity to take a journey like me, go within yourself, rediscover your power of communication and take charge of your internal monologue. By doing this, you learn to express your thoughts more effectively so that your thoughts, words, and actions can be powerful enough to create results in the world. Effective communication is beyond learning how to talk. It's about commanding the forces within you and others to create a favorable outcome. Healing begins in the mind, as you learn in this book. The program will show you how to manifest it.

NOTES

Part One

Aghanya, N. T. (2021). *Effective Communication Guidebook for Patients*. TAFFD's Publishers.

Kwik, J. (2020). *Limitless*. Hay House Inc.

Chukwu, U. A. (2020). *An Exercise in Clear Thinking: 11 Rules for Interpreting the World* (1st ed., Ser. 1). TAFFD's Publishers.

Fonda, A. (2015, February 13). Can we measure (physical) energy emitted from thoughts? Quora. https://www.quora.com/Can-we-measure-physical-energy-emitted-from-thoughts.

Markowsky, G. (n.d.). Physiology. Encyclopædia Britannica. https://www.britannica.com/science/information-theory/Physiology.

Reader, S. (2015, September 10). Conscious vs subconscious processing power. Speed Reading Courses London UK. https://spdrdng.com/posts/conscious-vs-subconscious-processing.

Sapolsky, R. M. (2020, December 30). The teenage brain: Why some years are (a lot) crazier than others. Big Think. https://bigthink.com/videos/what-age-is-brain-fully-developed.

Herndon, J. (2020, March 24). Vaginismus: Symptoms, Causes, Treatments, and More. Healthline. https://www.healthline.com/health/vaginismus#types.

Cafasso, J. (2018, July 18). How Many Cells Are in the Human Body? Types, Production, Loss, More. Healthline. https://www.healthline.com/health/number-of-cells-in-body#:~:text=Humans%20are%20complex%20organisms%

20made,Written%20out%2C%20that's%2030%2C000%2C00

0%2C000%2C000!

Hirsch, L. (Ed.). (2019, May). Brain and Nervous System (for

Teens) - Nemours KidsHealth. KidsHealth.

https://kidshealth.org/en/teens/brain-nervous-

system.html#:~:text=The%20brain%20controls%20what%2

0you,controls%20all%20the%20body's%20functions.

Khan Academy. (n.d.). Apoptosis (article) | Developmental

biology. Khan Academy.

https://www.khanacademy.org/science/biology/developme

ntal-biology/apoptosis-in-development/a/apoptosis.

Wikimedia Foundation. (2021, May 10). Hypoplasia.

Wikipedia. https://en.wikipedia.org/wiki/Hypoplasia.

Osteraas, N. D., & Lee, V. H. (2017, February 7).

Neurocardiology. Handbook of Clinical Neurology.

https://www.sciencedirect.com/science/article/pii/B978044

4636003000040#:~:text=Neurocardiology%20refers%20to%

20the%20interplay,injury%20that%20share%20oversympathe

tic%20activation.

SamuelsMD, M. A., Samuels, M. A., Martin A. Samuels From

the Department of Neurology, & Correspondence to Dr

Martin A. Samuels. (2007, July 3). The Brain–Heart

Connection. Circulation.

https://www.ahajournals.org/doi/10.1161/CIRCULATION

AHA.106.678995.

AM;, A. (n.d.). Pain: Is It All in the Brain or the Heart?

Current pain and headache reports.

https://pubmed.ncbi.nlm.nih.gov/31728781/.

Part Two

Aghanya, N. T. (2021). *Effective Communication Guidebook for

Clinicians*. TAFFD's Publishers.

Copleston, F. (1994). *A history of philosophy*. Image Books,

Doubleday.

Chukwu, U. A. (2021). *Infinite Learning: Principles to help you learn, become and create anything.* TAFFD's Publisher.

Plato, Cooper, J. M., & Hutchinson, D. S. (1997). *Plato: complete works.* Hackett.

Wikimedia Foundation. (2021, July 5). *Mass communication.* Wikipedia. https://en.wikipedia.org/wiki/Mass_communication.

Juárez Olguín, H., Calderón Guzmán, D., Hernández García, E., & Barragán Mejía, G. (2015, December 6). *The Role of Dopamine and Its Dysfunction as a Consequence of Oxidative Stress.* Oxidative Medicine and Cellular Longevity. https://www.hindawi.com/journals/omcl/2016/9730467/#:~:text=Dopamine%20is%20a%20neurotransmitter%20that,and%20hypothalamus%20of%20the%20brain.

Sathyanarayana Rao, T. S., Asha, M. R., Jagannatha Rao, K. S., & Vasudevaraju, P. (2009). *The biochemistry of belief.* Indian journal of psychiatry. https://www.ncbi.nlm.nih.gov/pmc/articles/PMC2802367/.

Which system in our brain controls our facial expressions during Bell's palsy? Crystal Touch Bell's Palsy Clinic. (2021, March 3). https://crystal-touch.nl/system-in-our-brain-that-controls-our-facial-expressions-during-bells-palsy/.

Eliscu, R. (2018, June 29). *Is the limbic system part of the nervous system or a separate system on its own?* Quora. https://www.quora.com/Is-the-limbic-system-part-of-the-nervous-system-or-a-separate-system-on-its-own.

Boundless. (n.d.). *Boundless Psychology*. Lumen. https://courses.lumenlearning.com/boundless-psychology/chapter/biology-of-emotion/#:~:text=Neurochemicals%20such%20as%20dopamine%2C%20noradrenaline,in%20response%20to%20emotional%20cues.

Authors Jessica Madrid. (n.d.). *Pupils: A Window Into the Mind.* Frontiers for Young Minds. https://kids.frontiersin.org/articles/10.3389/frym.2019.00003.

Germani, F. (2020, November 16). *Plato teaches us about scientific communication*. Culturico. https://culturico.com/2020/07/14/plato-teaches-us-about-scientific-communication/.

Team, T. F. (2020, December 3). *What's a Linear Model of Communication?* Fleximize. https://fleximize.com/articles/000561/a-linear-model-of-communication.

Five Types of Communication. Goodwin College of Professional Studies. (n.d.). https://drexel.edu/goodwin/professional-studies-blog/overview/2018/July/Five-types-of-communication/.

4 Types of Communication and How to Improve Them. Indeed Career Guide. (n.d.). https://www.indeed.com/career-advice/career-development/types-of-communication.

Tony DeFranco, T. C. C. (n.d.). *Principles of Management*. Lumen. https://courses.lumenlearning.com/atd-tc3-management/chapter/different-types-of-communication/.

Take Online Courses. Earn College Credit. Research Schools, Degrees & Careers. Study.com | Take Online Courses. Earn College Credit. Research Schools, Degrees & Careers. (n.d.). https://study.com/academy/lesson/what-are-the-different-levels-of-communication.html.

Young, L., & Saxe, R. (2008). The neural basis of belief encoding and integration in moral judgment. *neuroimage*, *40*(4), 1912-1920.

Five Levels of Communication. Scott Jeffrey. (2020, February 18). https://scottjeffrey.com/five-levels-of-communication/.

Part Three

Aghanya, N. T. (2021). *Principles for Overcoming Communication Anxiety and Improving Trust.* TAFFD's Publishers.

Aghanya, N. T. (2021). *Tips for Effective Communication: A Vital Tool for Trust Development in Healthcare .* TAFFD's Publishers.

Dispenza, J. (2015). *You are the placebo: making your mind matter.* Hay House, Inc.

Kalu, O. A. (2021). *Conquering the Beast Fear: A Philosophical Cum Psychological Approach.* TAFFD's Publisher.

Kalu, O. A. (2021). *The First Stage of the Fearologist: The Fearologist* (Vol. 1). TAFFD's Publisher's.

Kalu, O. A. (2021). *Success Mantra: Decoding Philosophy to a Purposeful Life.* TAFFD's Publisher.

Kalu, O. A., Subba, D., & Adhikari, B. S. (2020). *EcoFearism: Prospects & Burning Issues.* KDP Amazon.

Wikimedia Foundation. (2021, June 30). *Healing.* Wikipedia. https://en.wikipedia.org/wiki/Healing.

Jodi Clarke, M. A. (2021, February 12). *What to Know About the Five Stages of Grief.* Verywell Mind. https://www.verywellmind.com/five-stages-of-grief-4175361.

Salisbury, D. (1970, October 3). *Cell signals that trigger wound healing are surprisingly complex.* Vanderbilt University.

https://news.vanderbilt.edu/2017/10/03/cell-signals-that-trigger-wound-healing-are-surprisingly-complex/.

Salisbury, D. (1970, October 3). *Cell signals that trigger wound healing are surprisingly complex.* Vanderbilt University.

https://news.vanderbilt.edu/2017/10/03/cell-signals-that-trigger-wound-healing-are-surprisingly-complex/.

Lawhead, W. F. (2015). *The voyage of discovery: a historical introduction to philosophy.* Cengage Learning.

RM;, S. R. L. M. G. A. N. K. E. (n.d.). *How does communication heal? Pathways linking clinician-patient communication to health outcomes.* Patient education and counseling.

https://pubmed.ncbi.nlm.nih.gov/19150199/.

Salisbury, D. (1970, October 3). *Cell signals that trigger wound healing are surprisingly complex.* Vanderbilt University.

https://news.vanderbilt.edu/2017/10/03/cell-signals-that-trigger-wound-healing-are-surprisingly-complex/.

Five Levels of Communication. Scott Jeffrey. (2020, February 18).

https://scottjeffrey.com/five-levels-of-communication/.

Energy Balance Healing. therapies. (n.d.).

https://www.lizflynn.com/energy-balance-healing.

SUGGESTED READING

Aghanya, N. T. (2021). *Effective Communication Guidebook for Clinicians*. TAFFD's Publishers.

Aghanya, N. T. (2021). *Effective Communication Guidebook for Patients*. TAFFD's Publishers.

Aghanya, N. T. (2021). *Principles for Overcoming Communication Anxiety and Improving Trust*. TAFFD's Publishers.

Aghanya, N. T. (2021). *Tips for Effective Communication: A Vital Tool for Trust Development in Healthcare* . TAFFD's Publishers.

Candace Pert. *Molecules of emotion: Why you feel the way you feel.* New York, USA:

Chukwu, U. A. (2020). *An Exercise in Clear Thinking: 11 Rules for Interpreting the World* (1st ed., Ser. 1). TAFFD's Publishers.

Subba, D. (2014). *Philosophy of Fearism: Life is Conducted Directed and Controlled by Fear.* KDP Amazon.

Scribner Publications; 2003. ISBN-10: 0684846349. [Google Scholar]

Copleston, F. (1994). *A history of philosophy.* Image Books, Doubleday.

Ornstein R, Sobel D. *The healing brain: Breakthrough discoveries about how the brain keeps us healthy.* USA: Malor Books; 1999. ISBN-10: 1883536170. [Google Scholar]

Robbins A. *Unlimited power: The new science of personal excellence.* UK: Simon and Schuster; 1986. ISBN 0-7434-0939-6. [Google Scholar]

Braden G. *The spontaneous healing of belief.* Hay House Publishers (India) Pvt. Ltd; 2008. ISBN 978-81-89988-39-5. [Google Scholar]

Chopra D. *Ageless body, timeless mind: The quantum alternative to growing old. Hormony* Publishers; 1994. ISBN -10: 0517882124. [Google Scholar]

Lipton B. *The biology of belief: Unleashing the power of consciousness, matter and miracles.* Mountain of Love Publishers; 2005. ISBN 978-0975991473. [Google Scholar]

Bogousslavsky J, Inglin M. *Beliefs and the brain.* Eur Neurol. 2007;58:129–32. [PubMed] [Google Scholar]

Gundersen L. *Faith and healing.* Ann Intern Med. 2000;132:169–72. [PubMed] [Google Scholar]

Kwik, J. (2020). *Limitless.* Hay House Inc.

Kalu, O. A. (2021). *Conquering the Beast Fear: A Philosophical Cum Psychological Approach.* TAFFD's Publisher.

Mueller PS, Plevak DJ, Rummans TA. *Religious involvement, spirituality, and medicine: Implications for clinical practice.* Mayo Clin Proc. 2001;76:1225–35. [PubMed] [Google Scholar]

Patel AD, Peretz I, Tramo M, Labreque R. *Processing prosodic and musical patterns: A neuropsychological investigation. Brain Lang.* 1998;61:123–44. [PubMed] [Google Scholar]

Plato, Cooper, J. M., & Hutchinson, D. S. (1997). *Plato: complete works.* Hackett.

Tramo MJ. Biology and music. Music of the hemispheres. Science. 2001;291:54–6. [PubMed] [Google Scholar]

Young L, Saxe R. *The neural basis of belief encoding and integration in moral judgment. Neuroimage.* 2008;40:1912–20. [PubMed] [Google Scholar]

Aichhorn M, Perner J, Weiss B, Kronbichler M, Staffen W, Ladurner G. *Temporo-parietal junction activity in theory-of-mind tasks:* Falseness, beliefs, or attention. J Cogn Neurosci. 2009;21:1179–92. [PubMed] [Google Scholar]

Abraham A, Rakoczy H, Werning M, von Cramon DY, Schubotz RI. *Matching mind to world and vice versa: Functional dissociations between belief and desire mental state processing.* Soc Neurosci. 2009;1:18. [PubMed] [Google Scholar]

Saxe R. *Why and how to study Theory of Mind with fMRI. Brain Res.* 2006;1079:57–65. [PubMed] [Google Scholar]

Krummenacher P, Mohr C, Haker H, Brugger P. *Dopamine, paranormal belief, and the detection of meaningful stimuli.* J Cogn Neurosci. 2009 Jun 30; [Epub ahead of print] [PubMed] [Google Scholar]

Kalu, O. A. (2021). *Conquering the Beast Fear: A Philosophical Cum Psychological Approach.* TAFFD's Publisher.

Kalu, O. A. (2021). *The First Stage of the Fearologist: The Fearologist* (Vol. 1). TAFFD's Publisher's.

Kalu, O. A. (2021). *Success Mantra: Decoding Philosophy to a Purposeful Life.* TAFFD's Publisher.

Kalu, O. A., Subba, D., & Adhikari, B. S. (2020). *EcoFearism: Prospects & Burning Issues.* KDP Amazon.

Flannelly KJ, Koenig HG, Galek K, Ellison CG. *Beliefs, mental health, and evolutionary threat assessment systems in the brain.* J Nerv Ment Dis. 2007;195:996–1003. [PubMed] [Google Scholar]

Dispenza, J. (2015). *You are the placebo: making your mind matter.* Hay House, Inc.

Lawhead, W. F. (2015). *The voyage of discovery: a historical introduction to philosophy.* Cengage Learning.

www.ingramcontent.com/pod-product-compliance
Lightning Source LLC
Chambersburg PA
CBHW021142260726
48656CB00024B/1213